Community Care in Perspective

Community Care in Perspective

Care, Control and Citizenship

Edited by

John Welshman
Institute for Health Research, Lancaster University, UK
and

Jan Walmsley
School of Health and Social Welfare, The Open University, UK

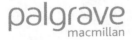

First published in 2006 by
PALGRAVE MACMILLAN
Houndmills, Basingstoke, Hampshire RG21 6XS and
175 Fifth Avenue, New York, N.Y. 10010
Companies and representatives throughout the world.

PALGRAVE MACMILLAN is the global academic imprint of the Palgrave
Macmillan division of St. Martin's Press, LLC and of Palgrave Macmillan Ltd.
Macmillan® is a registered trademark in the United States, United Kingdom
and other countries. Palgrave is a registered trademark in the European
Union and other countries.

ISBN-13: 978–1–4039–9265–9 hardback
ISBN-10: 1–4039–9265–7 hardback
ISBN-13: 978–1–4039–9266–6 paperback
ISBN-10: 1–4039–9266–5 paperback

This book is printed on paper suitable for recycling and made from fully
managed and sustained forest sources.

A catalogue record for this book is available from the British Library.

A catalog record for this book is available from the Library of Congress.

10 9 8 7 6 5 4 3 2 1
15 14 13 12 11 10 09 08 07 06

Printed and bound in Great Britain by
Antony Rowe Ltd, Chippenham and Eastbourne

Contents

v

Part IV   Experiences

Acknowledgements

We would particularly like to thank our editors at Palgrave, Philippa Grand and Jen Nelson; our referees at Palgrave; and Pat Chalk, Secretary to the Social History of Learning Disabilities (SHLD) Group at the Open University. John would like to acknowledge the funding provided through the OU's Associate Lecturer Development Fund, which helped with his travel to SHLD meetings. The Wellcome Trust funded some of his earlier work on the history of people with learning difficulties.

The authors and publishers have made every attempt to contact copyright holders. If any have inadvertently been overlooked, the appropriate arrangements will be made at the first opportunity.

John Welshman and Jan Walmsley

Notes on Contributors

Dorothy Atkinson is Professor of Learning Disability in the Faculty of Health and Social Care at the Open University. She was previously a social worker working with people with learning disabilities and their families, and her OU post involves research and teaching on current and past policies and practice. Her current research interests include oral and life history work with people with learning disabilities, their families and learning disability practitioners. She has co-edited a number of books on the history of learning disability, including *Forgotten Lives* (1997), *Crossing Boundaries* (2000) and *Witnesses to Change* (2005).

Rohhss Chapman works in the area of inclusive research and partnership with people with learning difficulties in Cumbria and closely with the self-advocacy movement. Her 2005 PhD thesis was about including people who receive services at all levels within organisations. Her current work includes an oral history project on the contributions and experiences of people with learning difficulties during the War years in Cumbria. She has written on inclusive research, partnership, and self-advocacy, and was a co-editor of *Witnesses to Change* (2005).

Kelley Johnson has worked for more than 15 years with people with learning difficulties in Australia. She has a particular interest in how people can lead good lives in the community, in working with women with disabilities, and in finding ways to include people with learning difficulties in research. She is a Senior Lecturer in Social Work at RMIT University in Melbourne, Australia, and is currently a Marie Curie Research Fellow at Trinity College, Dublin.

Sue Ledger has worked alongside people with learning difficulties in developing a range of support services in the UK, and with two overseas projects. She is particularly interested in Person Centred Planning and the design of person-centred teams, health inequalities, consent frameworks and the protection of vulnerable adults. She is currently completing her PhD with the Open University and is particularly interested in models of inclusive research and the use of video and multi media technology in life story work.

Duncan Mitchell is Professor of Health and Disability at Manchester Metropolitan University and Head of Clinical Services at Manchester

Learning Disability Partnership, the first holder of this joint appointment between the University and Partnership. Previously he was at the University of Salford where he was Head of the School of Nursing. He has also worked as a Community Learning Disability Nurse and has written on the history of learning disability.

Katherine Owen works as a qualitative researcher in the field of learning disability. She spent five years at St George's Hospital Medical School, where she carried out an ethnographic study of women with severe learning difficulties moving from a locked ward. Before that she worked as a support worker in both residential and day services, and completed an MA in Disability Studies at the University of Sheffield. She is currently doing a PhD at the Open University exploring people with learning difficulties' experiences of a Day Centre.

Sheena Rolph is a Senior Research Fellow in the Faculty of Health and Social Care at the Open University. Her research interests lie in the social history of learning disability, in particular the history of community care for people with learning difficulties in East Anglia. She has published on the history of Mental Welfare Officers; the ethics of oral history and archival research; aspects of the history of community care in East Anglia; the role of families in community care; and the history of local Mencap Societies. She recently completed two consecutive Heritage Lottery Funded projects on local Mencap Societies.

Tim Stainton is a former director of policy and programmes for the Ontario Association for Community Living. He is currently an Associate Professor of Disability Policy, Theory at the University of British Columbia. He is author of numerous works on disability rights, individualized funding, history, ethics and theory. His current research ranges between historical constructions of intellectual disability, ethics, models of individualized funding and service delivery, and disability rights.

Liz Tilley is completing her doctoral thesis in the Faculty of Health and Social Care at the Open University. Her research explores the growth of different types of advocacy organisations for people with learning difficulties, using a combination of historical and social science methods. Her broader research interests are around the historic and contemporary roles of voluntarism in the field of learning disability, and the interface between voluntary groups and the state.

Jan Tøssebro is Professor of Social Work at the Norwegian University of Science and Technology, Trondheim, Norway. His main areas of interest are deinstitutionalisation, inclusive education, families with disabled children, and living conditions of disabled people. He has served on Public Committees on disability policy and is currently chair of the Norwegian State Council on Disability. In English, he has among others co-edited the books *Intellectual Disabilities in the Nordic Welfare States* (1996), and *Exploring the Living Conditions of Disabled People* (2004).

James W. Trent is Professor of Sociology and Social Work at Gordon College, USA, and the author of *Inventing the Feeble Mind: A History of Mental Retardation in the United States* (1994).

Jan Walmsley is Visiting Professor of Learning Disability in the Faculty of Health and Social Care at the Open University. She is the author of *Inclusive Research in Learning Disability: Past Present and Futures*, as well as numerous papers, some of which relate to the history of learning disability which is her primary research interest.

John Welshman is Senior Lecturer in Public Health in the Institute for Health Research at Lancaster University. He is the author of *Underclass: A History of the Excluded, 1880–2000* (London and New York, 2006), and of recent articles in *Economic History Review*, the *Journal of Social Policy*, and *Twentieth Century British History*.

List of Abbreviations

APS	Adult Placement Scheme
ATC	Adult Training Centre
AWS	All Wales Strategy
CAMW	Central Association for Mental Welfare
CMH	Campaign for the Mentally Handicapped
ComSoc	Ministry of Community and Social Services (Canada)
CPS	Civilian Public Service (USA)
DAO	Duly Authorised Officer
DES	Department of Education and Science
DETR	Department of the Environment, Transport, and the Regions
DFEE	Department for Education and Employment
DHSS	Department of Health and Social Security
DHSSPS	Department of Health, Social Services and Public Safety (Northern Ireland)
DOH	Department of Health
ESEA	Elementary and Secondary Education Act (USA)
GPs	General Practitioners
HMC	Hospital Management Committee
HMSO	Her Majesty's Stationery Office
HRP	Homes for Retarded Persons Act (1966) (Canada)
HSC	Homes for Special Care Programme (Canada)
ICFs	Intermediate Care Facilities (USA)
IQ	Intelligence Quotient
JRF	Joseph Rowntree Foundation
JTC	Junior Training Centre
LEA	Local Education Authority
MOH	Medical Officer of Health
MWO	Mental Welfare Officer
NAMH	National Association for Mental Health
NAPBC	National Association of Parents of Backward Children
NARC	National Association for Retarded Children (USA)
NSMHCA	National Society for Mentally Handicapped Children and Adults
NCCL	National Council for Civil Liberties

NHS	National Health Service
OACL	Ontario Association for Community Living
OAMR	Ontario Association for the Mentally Retarded
OARC	Ontario Association for Retarded Children
PARC	Pennsylvania Association for Retarded Children
RHB	Regional Hospital Board
RO	Relieving Officer
SCIE	Social Care Institute of Excellence
SEC	Social Education Centre
SRV	social role valorisation
SSI	Supplemental Security Income (USA)
VRA	Vocational Rehabilitation Act (1966) (Canada)

Timeline: The UK in International Context

Year	UK	USA	Norway and Sweden	Canada	Australia
1943				Marsh Report on Social Security	
1944	Education Act				
1945					
1946	NHS Act	National Mental Health Foundation			
1947				First experimental school in Ontario for children with IQs under 50	
1948	NHS established	Albert Deutsch *The Shame of the States* *Forgotten Children: The Story of Mental Deficiency*			
1949				Pilot Programme in Toronto illustrating need for more classes for children	
1950	NCCL, *50,000 Outside the Law*	Pearl S. Buck, *The Child Who Never Grew*			
1951	Ministry of Health, *Report of the Committee on Social Workers* (MacIntosh Report)				
1952					
1953		Dale Evans Rogers, *Angel Unaware*		Formation of the OARC	

Continued

Continued

Year	UK	USA	Norway and Sweden	Canada	Australia
1954		US Supreme Court rules that 'separate is not equal'	Swedish Act on Education and Care for People with Learning Disabilities		
1955					
1956	O'Connor and Tizard, *The Social Problem of Mental Deficiency*				
1957	*Royal Commission on the Law Relating to Mental Illness and Mental Deficiency 1954–57*				
1958	Clarke and Clarke, *Mental Deficiency: The Changing Outlook*			First conference of the Canadian Association for Retarded Children	
1959	Mental Health Act (England and Wales) Ministry of Health, Department of Health for Scotland, *Report of the Working Party on Social Workers* (Younghusband Report)		Danish law text stated as a goal that people with learning disabilities should have the opportunity to 'live a life as close to normal as possible'	Report on Orillia in the *Toronto Star*	

Continued

Continued

Year	UK	USA	Norway and Sweden	Canada	Australia
1960	Jones, *Mental Health and Social Policy 1845–1959* Adams and Lovejoy, *The Mentally Subnormal*				
1961	Enoch Powell's 'water towers' speech	Erving Goffman, *Asylums* Thomas Szasz, *The Myth of Mental Illness* Gerald Caplan, *An Approach to to Community Mental Health*			
1962	Ministry of Health, *A Hospital Plan for England and Wales*	Eunice Kennedy Shriver article in the *Saturday Evening Post* Ken Kesey, *One Flew Over the Cuckoo's Nest*			
1963	Ministry of Health, *Health and Welfare: the Development of Community Care*	Mental Retardation Facilities and Community Mental Health Centers Construction Act			
1964	Tizard, *Community Services for the Mentally Handicapped*			Peak of Ontario's institution population	
1965		Senator Robert Kennedy critical of New York facilities			

Continued

Continued

Year	UK	USA	Norway and Sweden	Canada	Australia
1966		Burton Blatt and Fred Caplan, *Christmas in Purgatory*		Homes for Retarded Persons Act (Canada) Vocational Rehabilitation Act (Canada)	
1967	Ely Hospital, Cardiff, scandal	'Christmas in Purgatory', *Look* magazine Philippe de Broca's film, 'King of Hearts' Governor Ronald Reagan orders budget cuts in California Niels Bank-Mikkelsen critical of conditions in the Sonoma State Hospital, California	White Paper in Norway claims that the family can provide better care than any institution Norwegian film director compares residential schools to concentration camps Ombudsman concludes that residential schools are not appropriate for children Revised Service Act in Sweden		
1968	*Report of the Committee on Local Authority and Allied Personal Social Services* (Seebohm Report)				
1969	*Report of the Committee of Inquiry into Allegations of Ill-Treatment and Other Irregularities* (Howe Report) Morris, *Put Away* Numbers in institutions peaked				

Continued

Continued

Year	UK	USA	Norway and Sweden	Canada	Australia
1970	Education (Handicapped Children) Act		Number of residents of institutions peaked in Sweden and Denmark		
1971	Establishment of Social Services Departments (England and Wales) Establishment of Social Work Departments (Scotland) DHSS White Paper, *Better Services for the Mentally Handicapped* Report of the *Farleigh Hospital Committee of Inquiry* (Watkins Report) Oswin, *The Empty Hours* Baranyay, *The Mentally Handicapped Adolescent*			Martel and Sanderson tragedies Williston Report Wolf Wolfensberger begins term as visiting scholar at the National Institute for Mental Retardation, Toronto	
1972		Geraldo Rivera, 'Willowbrook: The Last Disgrace' Jane Mercer, 'IQ: The Lethal Label', *Psychology Today*			
1973	Clarke and Clarke, *Mental Retardation and Behavioural Research*	Education for all Handicapped Children Act	Norway Public Committee Report	Green Paper *Community Living for the Mentally Retarded: A New Policy Focus*	

Continued

Continued

Year	UK	USA	Norway and Sweden	Canada	Australia
1974	Deacon, *Tongue Tied* Clarke and Clarke, *Mental Deficiency: The Changing Outlook* (3rd edn)			Developmental Services Act A New Mental Retardation Program for Ontario	
1975	DHSS White Paper, *Better Services for the Mentally Ill* Jones, *Opening the Door* Tizard, Sinclair, and Clarke, *Varieties of Residential Experience*				
1976			Number of residents of institutions peaked in Norway, Finland, and Iceland		
1977	Normansfield Hospital Enquiry				
1978	DES, *Special Educational Needs: A Report* (Warnock Report)				
1979	*Report of the Committee of Enquiry into Mental Handicap Nursing and Care* (Jay Report) Griffiths Report				
1980				Bill 82	
1981	Education Act DHSS White Paper, *Care in the Community* Carter, *Day Centres*		Swedish Public Committee Report	Third International Self-Advocacy Conference, Toronto	

Continued

Continued

Year	UK	USA	Norway and Sweden	Canada	Australia
1982				Canada Act	
1983					
1984	Registered Homes Act				
	People First founded, London				
1985			Norway Public Committee Report Swedish Parliament revises legislation on services for people with learning disabilities		
1986	Disabled Persons (Services, Consultation and Representation) Act	Fourth International Self-Advocacy Conference, Anchorage, Alaska			Intellectually Disabled Persons Services Act
					Guardianship and Administration Board Act
1987					
1988	Education Reform Act		Legislation in Norway		
1989	Children Act DHSS White Paper, *Government Objectives for Community Care*				Three Year Plan
1990	NHS and Community Care Act				
1991	Registered Homes Amendment Act				
1992					

Continued

Continued

Year	UK	USA	Norway and Sweden	Canada	Australia
1993	Education Act				
1994					
1995	Disability Discrimination Act				Intellectual Disability Services Task Force
1996	Education Act				
	Direct Payments Act				
1997	Welsh Assembly set up				
	DfEE Green Paper, *Excellence for all Children*				
1998	Good Friday (Belfast) Agreement DfEE White Paper, *Meeting SEN: A Programme for Action*				
1999					
2000	Scottish Executive, *The Same as You?*		Deadline for closure of institutions in Sweden		
2001	DOH White Paper, *Valuing People*				
	Special Educational Needs and Disability Act (SENDA)				
2002	Department of Health and Social Services, *Review of Mental Health and Learning Disabilities (Northern Ireland)*				State Disability Plan, 2002–12 (Victoria)

Continued

Continued

Year	UK	USA	Norway and Sweden	Canada	Australia
2003	Welsh Assembly, *Fulfilling the Promises*				
2004					
2005					
2006	Deadline for closure of institutions in England				Draft Disability Bill
2007				Deadline for closure of institutions in Ontario	

Introduction

Jan Walmsley and John Welshman

Introduction

This book sets out to tell the often quite dramatic story of how, in the relatively short period of 50 years, the fortunes of people with learning difficulties changed quite dramatically. It is primarily a story of what happened in the United Kingdom (UK), though Part III of the book addresses developments in other parts of the Western world, highlighting significant convergences.

In 1948, when the newly formed National Health Service (NHS) took over responsibility for the long-stay hospitals, highly negative imagery of people with learning difficulties predominated, accompanied by punitive policies which segregated people, whether in institutions or within their families. There had been relatively little movement in this negative imagery since the early years of the century, when eugenic campaigners had successfully managed to portray these people as 'a terrible danger to the race' and initiated a policy of, where possible, detaining them in institutions. Community care, care provided outside of institutions, was in most parts of the world rudimentary, unless within that term we include care by families. Most expenditure went on building, maintaining and staffing large asylums. The community provision that did exist was seen, not as a means of enabling people to be part of society, but as an adjunct to institutional care, to be used when hospital care was too expensive, when there were no places, and when families could not be trusted to care efficiently for their offspring (Walmsley and Rolph, 2001).

By 2001, the date we have selected as the end point of our story, the imagery was very different. This was the date, in England, of *Valuing People*, the first White Paper to address learning disability since 1971. It

1

identified independence, choice, rights and inclusion as the proper objects of policy. Community-based services were the means by which these were promoted, now firmly relocated outside the formal Health Services (DOH, 2001a). Furthermore, beyond the confines of Government policy, aspirations were being expressed for full citizenship. Local Parliaments of people with learning disabilities sprang up in the wake of *Valuing People* (Dearden-Phillips and Fountain, 2005). If the history of learning disability policy can be characterised as swings from pessimism to optimism (Stainton, 2000), the turn of the twenty-first century can be seen as the zenith of a period of optimism swelling with possibilities and promises of a better, fuller life for this most disadvantaged of groups.

In this book we explore this extraordinary historical transition. We examine community care, the growth of services which transmuted, at least in rhetoric, from an adjunct to the institution to the means for inclusion and rights. And we explore the shifting ground between drivers which emphasise care or control, rights or risk. We also take the opportunity to look beneath the surface through focusing not just on policy, but on experience, and the question of whether the surface changes were anything more than that. Have things really changed so dramatically for the majority of people with learning difficulties and their families, or are we looking at the promise of change without anything really being so different on a day-to-day basis for the majority of people so labelled?

Our distinctive approach

To effect our exploration of community care we take a distinctive approach which differs from most studies of policy change. Alongside the more traditional chapters describing the evolution of ideas (Part I), the changing organisations and structures supporting community care in the UK (Part II), and accounts from the USA, Scandinavia, Canada and Australia (Part III), we include a stakeholder approach, telling the story from the perspectives of different groups involved in the history of learning difficulties – families, voluntary sector organisations, staff and people who use the services (Part IV). We achieve this through use of life histories, oral histories and autobiographical approaches, alongside detailed archival research into documentary sources.

Life stories are a means of supplementing official history so that a further, more personal, dimension to historical issues is provided. Until recently, the perspectives of people with learning disabilities were ignored. Their symbolic and actual exclusion from ordinary, everyday life meant that they had frequently 'become invisible' (Bornat, 1992). As a consequence, outside the specialist field of learning disability little has been heard of their life experiences, adding further to the mystification of learning disability and providing opportunity for myths based on ignorance to be perpetuated. People with learning disabilities are particularly susceptible to being marginalised (Edge, 2001), excluded and treated as 'unreliable witnesses' (Craft, 1987) with little of interest to say (Atkinson, 1998b). Recently researchers such as Atkinson (1998b, Atkinson *et al.*, 2000a) and Goodley (1996) have argued that through the use of biographical and oral history methods we can begin to redress the balance, enabling these hidden voices (Atkinson and Walmsley, 1999) to be heard and a fuller history of learning disability to be recorded. Such accounts enable a wider audience to gain a clearer understanding of what it is like to live with the label of learning disability and be in receipt of services, or to live alongside a person with learning disabilities as a family member or close friend (Rolph *et al.*, 2005). We hope this book will support more readers to gain that insight. Recently the use of multi-media, theatre and memory boxes have enabled the inclusion in this process of people with learning disabilities who do not use speech to communicate. There has also been increased emphasis on documenting the life stories of those from minority groups (Downer and Ferns, 1998; Black Friendly Group, 2004) and those who remained at home with families rather than entering any form of institutional care (Walmsley, 1995b).

Through these more individualised accounts of people with learning disabilities, family members or close friends, people emerge not as deficient in skills or lacking the correct social behaviour, but as individuals with a personal history, culture, social class and gender in addition to the label (Atkinson and Williams, 1990). Life stories can cut through the stereotype of people with learning disabilities as passive victims of oppressive systems, by highlighting people's resistance against oppression and resilience in the face of adversity (Potts and Fido, 1991; Goodley, 1996). Finally, the construction of life stories can be important as a means by which people are empowered through the process of doing research (Atkinson, 1998b, 2002).

Drawing on this vein of research focusing on people's stories, the book allows an exploration of not only evolving ideas and policy makers' intentions, but also how policy impacted on people's lives – a much more difficult story to tell. The idea that there is a plurality of accounts which weave 'history' is a late twentieth-century phenomenon which replaced an earlier tradition, the search for the authoritative account. In

Jan's undergraduate days, in the late 1960s, history was not problematised in this way. Different historians had their own theories and ideas, but we owe it largely to feminism that there is now a recognition that what constitutes history is, to some extent, in the eye of the beholder. Sheila Rowbotham and her contemporaries-followers started a trend from which other groups have benefited – a trend that recognised that some groups have been left out of historical accounts, unseen players whose stories deserve consideration (Hall Carpenter Archives, 1989; Jewish Women in London Group, 1989).

The stakeholders whose stories are told in Part IV include people with learning disabilities, family members, the voluntary sector, professionals – social workers, nurses, psychiatrists, psychologists, managers – and front line workers such as those who staff day and residential facilities. This is a different list to that which can be readily accessed via conventional historians' source material – official papers, policy documents, diaries and biographies. To access the perspectives of these stakeholders the authors have drawn on oral accounts, some published works, particularly anthologies and documented reminiscence, letters, photograph albums, cine film, minute books of local Societies and other local archives. The authors are uniquely placed, having, through the work of the Social History of Learning Disability Group, been collecting such sources for the past 20 years. The Group's pioneering work includes life stories of people with learning difficulties (see, e.g., Cooper, 1997; Atkinson and Cooper, 2000), documented family reminiscence (Rolph *et al.*, 2005); research into the origins and achievements of local Mencap Societies (Rolph, 2002, 2005a–f); research into the operation of self-advocacy groups (Clement, 2004; Chapman, 2005; Tilley, forthcoming); alongside more substantive work on methodology (Walmsley, 1995a; Atkinson, 1998a); the history of learning disability nursing (Mitchell, 2000); and policy evolution and service delivery (Welshman, 1999a, 2000, 2006a).

This work is primarily UK-focused. However, the book aspires to give its readers a sense of the UK in international perspective, and includes chapters on developments in community care in key comparator countries (Part III). All these chapters are authored by local experts who, like the principal authors, espouse the view that the stories of those affected by major policy developments deserve consideration.

Why learning difficulties?

It may well be asked why privilege people with learning difficulties in telling the story of community care? After all, community care policies have impacted on all of society's vulnerable groups – older people, people with mental health problems and people with physical impairments. The reason for this is that such a history has not yet been written, whereas there have been thorough and scholarly socio-historical analyses of services outside asylums for other groups (Means and Smith, 1985; Pilgrim and Rogers, 1993; Means *et al.*, 2003). We would also tentatively suggest that the changes for people with learning difficulties have been startling and dramatic, more so than for any other group. In 1975, Kathleen Jones argued that the obstacles to progress were not primarily economic, but arose from the fact that the 'mentally handicapped' were a relatively small group in society, who could not compete for resources on their own behalf. But other reasons were particular to mental handicap itself:

> Some are lovable – that is, they elicit an easy response of protectiveness and affection. Some are harder to love ... some ... are unattractive in appearance ... Getting to know them is hard work. They are not 'grateful' for services and do not easily reciprocate gestures of friendship. Affection, if aroused, may take embarrassing and demanding forms. (Jones, 1975, pp. 202–4)

It is almost impossible to imagine such an analysis being published now, around 30 years later. Not only is legislation in place to outlaw the sorts of behaviours Jones describes, but there is a belief in people's rights to be regarded as fellow human beings. The commitments in *Valuing People* have set these out. A study of history can help us to probe behind current beliefs and taboos to find out where these changes in attitude have come from and what they mean.

People with learning difficulties: who are we talking about?

The book's title begs many questions. We have chosen to focus on 'people with learning difficulties' for the reasons explained above, but who are we talking about when we use this, often contested, term? The current definitions of learning disability by, for example, the British Psychological Society (2001) and the American Association on Mental Retardation (1992) use the dual criterion of low Intelligence Quotient (IQ) and maladaptive functioning. Yet, beyond some crude and often misused IQ categories, there is little consensus, other than a pragmatic definition that these are people in receipt of services associated with learning disability – Special Schools, Day Centres, etc. This is the approach we take in this book. However, relatively few people who can be predicted as having a learning disability-difficulty (commonly, as in *Valuing People*, estimated at 2.5 per cent of the population) are in receipt of services at any one time (Whitaker, 2004). And it needs to be noted that as policies change, so do the categories. A number of people with learning difficulties are buying their own homes through shared owner-ship schemes.[1] This is rightly seen as a marker of citizen status, a major breakthrough for people who more often live in someone else's house with little autonomy. However, as they become householders, their identity as people with learning difficulties becomes less clear. If they get support it is likely to be home care supplied by agencies which serve a range of client groups. They may well be in receipt of Disablement Allowance or Incapacity Benefit, but neither of these is specific to learn-ing disability. Thus, unless defined by their past as more traditional serv-ice users, they cease to be readily identifiable as people with learning difficulties. We have chosen to follow the example of other authors in defining people by their use of services, past or present. But it should also be noted that if policies relating to inclusion in mainstream schools and moving to a system of Direct Payments-individualised budgets for adults prevail – as is the current intention (DOH, 2005) – the approach we have taken will become even more problematic.

Categorisation poses other problems. The term 'people with learning difficulties' covers a wide spectrum of impairments and abilities, from people who are, with some gentle support, able to earn their own living, or at least live pretty independent lives, to people who require assistance with the most basic tasks of living – eating, moving, communicating. One of the dangers of the optimism associated with *Valuing People* is that people's needs can come to be minimised. Progress towards full citizen-ship has been considerable for a few, particularly more able people, whereas for the majority there continue to be problems associated with poverty, petty crime, bullying, name calling and harassment (Emerson *et al.*, 2005). As Johnson and Traustadottir put it: 'bricks and mortar are relatively easy to tear down and build. It is much more difficult to find ways of supporting people so that they can have meaningful lives that are akin to those of other citizens' (2005, p. 26).

The use of labels is another contentious area related to the people we are discussing. There are few groups for whom the approved terminol-ogy has changed so rapidly as in the period covered by our history. At the outset, in the 1940s, 'mental defective' was still being used, a term which entered the policy vocabulary before 1913. The 1959 Mental Health Act replaced this term with 'subnormal'. This term was in its turn replaced in the 1971 White Paper *Better Services for the Mentally Handicapped* with 'the mentally handicapped'. There followed a period of turbulent redefinitions, with 'people with a mental handicap' (as opposed to 'mentally handicapped people') rapidly followed by 'people with learning disabilities', adopted by the Department of Health (DOH) in the early 1990s, contrary to the stated preference of self-advocacy groups for 'people with learning difficulties', the term we have used, for political reasons, in this book. The terminology, in the UK at least, has remained relatively stable since the mid-1990s. Given the past decade has also been one of stability in the ideological stance taken by Government towards people with learning difficulties, it is tempting to argue that rapidly changing terminology is a reflection of policy and intellectual turbulence. At periods when positions become more fixed (as between 1913 and the 1950s, and possibly, since around 1993) then the terminology remains constant. Whatever the reasons for change and continuity in the labels we use, our practice is to respect historical usage, that is, we do not change terms where they clearly violate the intended meaning, but, where we refer to contemporary issues, as here, we use the term 'people with learning difficulties'. In so doing, we recognise the confusion this poses for international audiences, who not only use different terms (intellectual disability in Australia and New Zealand, developmental disabilities and mental retardation in the USA), but also use 'learning difficulties or disability' to mean difficulties with learning associated with, for example, dyslexia.

Furthermore, there is little doubt that not only the label but also those included in the category has changed over time. The 1913 Mental Deficiency Act included, alongside 'imbeciles, idiots' and 'feeble-minded', a category of 'moral defective', defined as people who from an early age displayed 'some permanent mental defect coupled with strong vicious or criminal propensities on which punishment had little or no effect' (Jones, 1960, p. 67). In practice, the 'moral defective' label could be, and was, used to detain individuals who were not intellectually challenged, but who did challenge the social order in some way (Cox, 1996; Walmsley, 2000b). We would argue, though not with total conviction, that such individuals are catered for by other means in the early twenty-first century, in pupil exclusion units, through Anti-Social Behaviour Orders, detention in the Youth Justice system, but rarely through being incorporated into services aimed at people with learning difficulties. Indeed, the shift of rhetoric from control to citizenship, which is a central theme of this book, makes the 'learning difficulties' label quite inappropriate for people who are constructed as threatening. The menace associated with mental defectives in early twentieth-century Britain has evaporated, or been attached to other groups (asylum seekers, people with personality disorder and so on), meaning, we suggest, that there is no direct correlation between early twentieth-century 'mental defectives' and those called 'people with learning difficulties' today.

Why community care and how do we define it?

We make community care a focus for very good reasons. Not only is community care the dominant policy framework within which learning disability services now sit in the countries of the UK, its history has also been a neglected area of study. We argue that throughout history, 'community care', if we include in that term care in families, has been the dominant mode of care provision for most people most of the time (Andrews, 1996). Notwithstanding this, the historiography of learning disability (and mental health) has been dominated by the institution (Bartlett and Wright, 1999). Institutions have physical presences which community alternatives often lack. Similarly they often have written records, while those of families, if they exist at all, are much more widely dispersed (Noll and Trent, 2004). Institutional lifestyles have attracted attention in part because they have been so different from 'normal' life, and stories of residents' suffering, abuse and resistance have been recorded and published (see, e.g., Potts and Fido, 1991; Cooper, 1997). Normalisation theories have been based on the abnormality of institutional life, where there is an implied contrast with normal life (Walmsley and Rolph, 2001). The result has been that life 'outside the walls of the asylum' has been neglected by historians. Recent work on the history of care in the community has revealed how families have always had an important role in care in the community, and how the boundaries between institutions and the community, and between the statutory and voluntary sectors have never been fixed (Thomson, 1998a; Wright, 1998; Bartlett and Wright, 1999; Walmsley, 2000a; Rolph, 2002).

Philip Abrams, writing in 1977, suggested that 'to those with a passion for conceptual tidiness the whole field of social care must be exceptionally frustrating; within that field community care is perhaps the least tidy corner' (Abrams, 1977, p. 125). Meanings and emphases continued to evolve significantly over the period under discussion. At the beginning of the period we address, community care was an adjunct to the institution. It then mutated as the alternative to the institution. At least before 1979, community care implied that Health Authorities and local authorities rather than families themselves should play the lead in providing care, and therefore in devising services and committing resources to this objective. This assumes the provision of publicly funded community services as the key to community care. But private care offers a cheap alternative to publicly funded and provided services, and, from the mid-1970s, community care has been reinterpreted from the development of public community services to that of private care in the community (Busfield, 1986, pp. 349–50), an adjunct not to the institution but to family-provided care. More recently, community care has moved further to an ideal type where the client becomes the consumer, choosing to spend his or her money, provided by the state, on the goods and services of his or her choosing, the individualised payments model, while being helped into employment. This is the model most closely associated with citizenship. We do not view any of these different formulations as necessarily better than the others, but we do try to locate them within their proper historical contexts.

As if difficulties with defining our subjects, and how to refer to them, were not enough, community care itself has been subject to numerous attempts at definition (see Means, *et al.*, 2003). The central argument in the book is that community care shifted in meaning during the period under discussion, from an undesirable but necessary *adjunct* to institutional care to be used when no institutional places were available (Walmsley and Rolph, 2001) to a positive *alternative* which conjured up images of belonging to the mainstream, ultimately itself to be dislodged in favour of 'social care' (DOH, 2005) an equally ill-defined and flexible term encompassing a wide range of provision including 'services which help support people in their daily lives and let them play a full part in society ... practical assistance to help individuals overcome barriers to inclusion ... support in managing complex relationships and emotional distress' (Taylor, 2006, p. 38).

The details of the debate on 'community care' which explain some of the confusion associated with it are explored in more depth in Part I 'Ideology and Ideas', and only a flavour of this debate is covered here. In the index to her 1960 study, for example, Kathleen Jones included under 'community care' 'day hospitals, half-way houses, night hospitals, mental aftercare, mental health departments, outpatient clinics, trichotomy' (Jones, 1960). Writing in 1994, on the other hand, Wright, Haycox and Leedham noted that policy was:

> very much in terms of providing community based care that gives people with learning difficulties opportunities to experience as full a

life as possible within the communities in which they live ... People with learning difficulties should maintain as normal a life as possible, should develop life skills to a personal maximum capacity and should be integrated into, not segregated from, the general life of the community. (pp. 4–5)

The term 'community care' itself is now becoming part of the past, discarded in favour of the term 'social care', possibly because the latter is a broader term encompassing social exclusion as well as the groups traditionally associated with care services (Taylor, 2006). This illustrates a particular problem with writing such recent history. We are, most of us, familiar with community care as 'news' items in newspapers, magazines like *Community Care* itself, television and radio programmes. When does this familiar news become history, part of the past? We set 2001 as the end date, a mere three years before the inception of the writing of the book. As we sat down to write it we were acutely aware that we were about to chronicle large chunks of our own lives as 'history'. Not only that, because it is so recent, much of it, there are plenty of people around who have their own memories. We hope that readers will bring to the story we tell their own experiences and memories, to augment and challenge the picture we paint. Since history is not one story, but many, coloured by the different experiences different stakeholders bring to bear on the telling, readers should find their own individual experiences reflected in at least some of the book's chapters.

Care, control and citizenship

The final set of definitions relates to 'care', 'control' and 'citizenship' which are the terms we believe best enable examination of the nature and purpose of care services in the period under discussion. As we set out to write the book, we had in our minds a fairly straightforward trajectory which saw services in 1948 being about control, gradually shading into 'care' with *Better Services*, and shifting from then to the end of the century towards a citizenship model. This may well describe national policy intentions reasonably accurately, but as we got into the grain of survivors' accounts, and in-depth contemporary studies we realised that it is a far more nuanced picture (Jones, 1975; Carter, 1981).

Where we use 'control' as a descriptor of service provision we refer to services which are overtly intended to protect society from the individual, whether by keeping him or her detained, or by preventing reproduction, often both. It is easy to characterise early twentieth-century mental deficiency policy as primarily motivated by control, though there was always a strand of protection, even in the most eugenically dark periods (Walmsley, 2005). Mary Dendy, a leading campaigner for institutional care in the early twentieth-century, for example, mentioned protecting the individual from society as one of the five reasons for permanent institutional care (Dendy, 1903; Jackson, 2001), and there is plentiful evidence that people were admitted to institutions because of family abuse or neglect (Rolph and Walmsley, 2006). One of our key arguments is that community care had existed throughout the twentieth century as an adjunct to institutions. Such services were as much about control as about care. This runs counter to the view, commonly expressed until relatively recently, that community care replaced institutional care as the dominant policy framework, and that this was influenced by more enlightened views about the potential of people with learning difficulties. Although the legal framework of the Mental Deficiency Acts vanished in 1959, it is unwise to regard community care as essentially more benign than institutional care. Much depends on how it is implemented.

Care, on the other hand, refers to services which are motivated by a desire to protect and support. But complications arise because even the most controlling services are needed to supply basic physical care – feeding, cleaning, clothing – and in the 1970s this was all many care services provided, even though the rhetoric was about development and potential (DHSS, 1971; Oswin, 1971; Jones, 1975). In 1981 Carter showed that although development and potential were in the lexicon of aims for Day Centres for people with learning difficulties, the practice was very different and they were in danger of becoming 'little more than big buildings in which the mentally handicapped are protected from the outside world' (Carter, 1981, p. 58). Similarly, Maureen Oswin's accounts of life for children in long-stay hospitals show that while their physical needs were met, their emotional and development needs were neglected. A philosophy of care amounted to little other than physical care (Oswin, 1971). Aspirations mean little when translated into day to day practices which accord to the individual little autonomy or opportunity for relationships and meaningful activity.

Whereas one might argue that services for people with learning difficulties have always danced around the twin poles of care and control, citizenship is the latecomer. The aspiration for citizenship is most noticeably expressed in *Valuing People*. In the accessible version

(DOH, 2001b) it simply states that 'people with learning disabilities are citizens too' (p. 3). The full version states that:

> People with learning disabilities have the right to a decent education, to grow up to vote, to marry and have a family and to express their opinions, with help and support to do so where necessary ... All public services will treat people with learning disabilities as individuals with respect for their dignity, and challenge discrimination on all grounds including disability. People with learning disabilities will also receive the full protection of the law when necessary. (DOH, 2001a, p. 23)

The full version does not actually use the term 'citizens' as does the accessible version, rather spells out what 'enforceable civil rights' might mean – decent education, voting, marrying and having a family, expressing opinions, being treated with dignity and having protection under the law.

The implications of a citizenship agenda for marginalised groups have been the subject of considerable discussion (Rioux *et al.*, 1997). Suffice it to say here that without action to address systematic inequalities, a commitment to rights is inadequate. It is not our intention at this point in the book to consider how far this aspiration has been achieved, nor to speculate on whether these are adequate aspirations, rather to note that here we have an emphasis which was missing from previous policy relating to this group, a policy which, alongside other principles of *Valuing People* – 'promoting independence', making choices and inclusion – distinguish it from any of its predecessors, and fully justifies the emphasis we give citizenship as a theme of the book.

Key themes

In developing the book we have identified certain themes which can help the reader make sense of the history. These themes appear to transcend national boundaries, as is evidenced by the four international perspectives:

- Historically care in the community has been as much about control as care
- The shift from institutional care to community care as the preferred 'solution' to the challenges presented by learning disability was roughly simultaneous across a number of countries, prompted by ideological change, revelations of abuse in institutions and economic considerations

- The debate about the proper intention of services has rhetorically moved from care and control to rights and citizenship, though the reality of the latter for many is far removed
- The advent of an organised parents' movement can be regarded as possibly the most significant development of the second half of the twentieth century in a number of Western countries
- The service user movement, self-advocacy, has had a significant though inconsistent impact on policy
- There have been, and continue to be, significant local variations in the way community care has been implemented.

The structure of the book

The book opens (Part I) with a consideration of how ideology and ideas underpinned the shift to community care. Part II addresses the organisations and structures which supported community care. For this purpose the period is divided into two, with a watershed in 1971 with *Better Services*. A separate chapter addresses changes in Scotland, Wales and Northern Ireland as, since UK devolution, policies have diverged increasingly. Part III consists of four chapters giving an international perspective on the development of community care in the Western world. The USA, Scandinavia (particularly Norway and Sweden), Ontario in Canada and Victoria in Australia are covered, all authored by distinguished local experts. The chapters in Part IV are authored by members of the Social History of Learning Disability Group at the Open University. They are accounts of the history of the period from the perspectives of different stakeholders, and draw extensively, but by no means exclusively, on oral accounts. Finally, the Conclusion draws together the main themes and findings to emerge from the book as a whole.

Note

1. Neil Morris personal communication, 2005.

Part I

Ideology and Ideas

Part I of the book explores the evolution of ideas which have helped to change perceptions of learning disability, from a problem of control to one of promoting citizenship and inclusion. The first chapter examines how changing ideas, accompanied by empirical research, created a platform for the discrediting of institutions as the preferred policy option, and explores the various conceptualisations of care in the community. The second chapter describes the impact of normalisation and the social model of disability on the way disability is conceived in policy terms, and how the image of people with learning disabilities has altered. By the end of the twentieth century, leading thinkers argued that people with learning difficulties are people who should have equal rights with others (citizens).

1
Ideology, Ideas and Care in the Community, 1948–71

John Welshman

Introduction

To understand the changes over the period we are examining, with dramatic policy shifts from institutional segregation to integration, then from integration to inclusion and citizenship, it is important to examine changes in ideology. In this chapter, the focus is particularly upon ideologies that led to the discrediting of the types of solutions adopted in the early part of the century – segregation, exclusion and control – and the adoption of policies with care as their central *leitmotif*. Dates have ideological significance. The year 1944 saw an Education Act in which, according to Sheena Rolph, 'many of the worst aspects of the [eugenic] ideology were enshrined in legislation; segregation, "ascertainment" and the concept of "ineducability".' (2005a–f, p. 14). In 1948 the NHS was founded, which took responsibility for mental deficiency institutions from local authorities, voluntary organisations and private providers, signalling the dominance of a medical model. At the end of the period these trends were to an extent reversed. In 1970 the Education Act gave all children the right to an education, and 1971 saw *Better Services* which is seen as a landmark in the move to community care, and signalled the end (though very slow) of the NHS's control of services. We can see the early 1970s as a watershed, the time when policy makers adopted the relatively optimistic ideas associated with researchers who made the case for regarding people with mental handicaps as able to benefit from a comfortable environment, contact with the wider world and education.

It is, however, important to acknowledge that ideas alone do not drive change – though they can influence the direction of changes. The difference between what is said and done underlies our decision to separate

17

the analysis of ideological change from the account of changes in organisations and structures, which are covered in Part II of the book. We can characterise the view of people with learning difficulties in 1948 as one in which their passivity and neediness were unquestioned. They were seen as people who needed physical care and control, either within institutions or carefully policed within their families on the basis of an unchanging and unchangeable individualised pathology (Burt, 1952; Lyons and Heaton-Ward, 1955). By the end of the 1960s this view was being challenged from a number of quarters – by psychologists like Jack Tizard who argued for a much more dynamic view of people's potential; by sociologists like Goffman who pointed to the negative impact of institutionalisation; and, probably most importantly, by families who, banded together in voluntary organisations like the National Society for Mentally Handicapped Children and Adults (NSMHCA) (later Mencap), demanded community-based services, support and recognition of their children as human beings (Rolph *et al.*, 2005). The impact of this ideological shift on policy can be characterised from one broadly concerned with control, to one more focused on issues of care (Walmsley and Rolph, 2001).

We argue that these changing ideas were reflected in the changing views of what constitutes 'community care', from services which are primarily an adjunct to institutional care, to be used as a regrettable last resort, to the provision of a set of services spatially placed nearer to centres of population, ideas reflected in *Better Services*. Notwithstanding these changes, it needs to be noted that institutional populations peaked in 1969, indeed were almost twice as high as in 1948, and new hospitals continued to be built. There is a long timelag between ideas and implementation. The chapter will seek to chart the ideological changes. How far and how quickly they were implemented are dealt with in Part II.

Control, eugenics and mental deficiency

We open our discussion with a brief consideration of the ideology prevailing at the beginning of our period, eugenics. As noted above, ideas associated with eugenics were still entering into legislation as late as the 1944 Education Act. Furthermore, the legislation most closely associated with eugenics, the Mental Deficiency Act passed in 1913, with its emphasis on segregation in institutions, and careful control of those remaining in the community, remained the legislative framework until 1959. Eugenic ideas about the need to control defective and feeble-minded children and adults are the starting point against which we can set the shift in the 1950s to ideas that were arguably more about care (*Report of the Royal Commission*, 1908; Walmsley and Rolph, 2001). Eugenic ideas always comprised elements of care, although control was paramount. Early twentieth-century campaigners such as Mary Dendy, for example, argued that permanent segregation of the feeble-minded had benefits, both for society at large and for the individuals segregated (Dendy, 1903; Jackson, 2001). Permanent care was both scientific and moral. Jackson shows how the feeble-minded were represented as pathological and distinct from the normal population, because it was believed they were incurable educationally and socially inept. This, in turn, was used to legitimise claims that the only rational solution was permanent segregation. Colonies might be situated in sparsely populated areas and should aim at a 'simple wholesome life' where the inmates were 'happy and harmless'. The twin aims of care and control were always present, but control was a far more prominent driver than care. The prominent eugenist A. F. Tredgold wrote in 1909 that 'colony life would at the same time protect the feeble-minded against a certain section of society and protect society against the feeble-minded' (Tredgold, 1909, pp. 97–104).

Eugenics led to an essentially pessimistic view of the potential of 'mental defectives'. Under the 1913 Act, of the four groups that were created, idiots and imbeciles were regarded as definitely ineducable; whereas the feeble-minded and moral imbeciles could be labelled as ineducable after trial. All groups were to be segregated from others, and local authorities were expected to identify ('ascertain') all defectives and to provide institutional care. Children were either excluded from school or, for a minority, placed in Special Schools or classes. Only in 1970 under the Education (Handicapped Children) Act were some 24,000 children returned to the care of the general educational system (Gabbay and Webster, 1983). In the 1920s and 1930s, anxieties about mental deficiency were prominent in the construction of the 'social problem group', and debates around the relative merits of a policy of sterilisation was evidence of an explicit control agenda relating to mental deficiency. The key event in spreading the concept of the social problem group was the Report of the Mental Deficiency Committee (1929). The most important aspect of the Report was the alleged increase in the incidence of mental deficiency (Board of Education and Board of Control, 1929, part 3, paras 96–102). In terms of prevention, the options were segregation and sterilisation. The key problem identified was that the families of the 'subnormal' group remained large, while families of the 'better' social groups were becoming smaller.

Following the publication of the Wood Report, the Eugenics Society intensified its efforts in support of a policy of sterilisation, and it sought to build a coalition of support among the social work, mental health and public health professions. Public meetings in support of sterilisation were held up to the outbreak of the Second World War (Macnicol, 1989, pp. 154–9; King, 1999, p. 72). However, in the UK, unlike in a number of European countries, and many US states, the campaign for legalised sterilisation of mental defectives was not successful. The Catholic church opposed the idea on ideological grounds as did the Labour Party, and the proposed sterilisation programme was damaged from January 1934 by revelations of the Nazi campaign of compulsory sterilisation and euthanasia (Jones, 1986). By the late 1930s, various factors were combining to weaken the legitimacy of eugenics and sterilisation. The mood of crisis that had characterised the early 1930s had evaporated by the latter half of the decade, as the economy began to recover, and the social and political fabric had shown itself to be strong enough to withstand the strains to which it had been subjected. Demographic investigations were destroying the foundations of many eugenic theories, such as the phenomenon of the differential birth rate. Eugenics was increasingly under attack from scientists such as Lancelot Hogben, and research, such as that of John Boyd Orr on nutrition, directed attention more to environmental than hereditarian factors. In particular, an emerging Keynesian middle-way consensus was holding out an optimistic and convincing strategy for non-socialist reformism. In this context, many began to argue that environmental reform was a complementary component of eugenics (Searle, 1981, pp. 150–69; Kevles, 1995, pp. 164–75; Macnicol, 1987, p. 313).

The situation in 1948

In 1948, it would be hard to argue that there was a major ideological shift. Rather, the placing of the services in the NHS indicates an assumption that mental deficiency was a medical problem best addressed by placing doctors and nurses in charge (Richardson, 2005). News of the Nazis' extermination practices appears to have been influential in discrediting sterilisation (Jones, 1986). But there was no discernible intellectual challenge to the assumptions underpinning institutionalisation as the optimum treatment, or to the segregation of the sexes intended to prevent 'breeding' by defectives (Humphries and Gordon, 1992; Gelb, 2004). Indeed, it is quite remarkable, that, since Wedgwood's challenge in 1913 on the grounds of liberty of the subject, there had been no fundamental opposition to the precepts of the 1913 Act for over 30 years, resistance being confined to further draconian proposals such as marriage bans and enforced sterilisation (Stainton, 1992, p. 20, 2000). Eugenically inspired enquiries into the causes of social problems continued into the 1940s, and there is plentiful evidence in local records of a continuity of an attitude which characterised mental defectives as a threat to society.[1]

It was outside the mainstream of service provision that change in thinking is noticeable. The most important development was arguably the founding of the first branches of the National Society for Parents of Backward Children (NSPBC). Its story is told in detail in Chapters 11 and 14. Prewar voluntary organisations were not stakeholder bodies – postwar saw the development of stakeholder membership groups which campaigned for fundamental changes. It would be hard to overstate the importance of this development, so characteristic of postwar voluntary organisations, but virtually unknown prior to that. The 'why then' question is important, but its answer unclear. Rolph cites the coming of the welfare state as one of the key influences, because it raised expectations: 'the realisation that children excluded from school were also excluded from free meals, free milk and supplements, and were not eligible for family allowances, caused much resentment among parents' (Rolph, 2002, p. 26). However, as the chapters in Part III show, this phenomenon was not confined to countries with welfare states. The USA, where there was no welfare state, also saw parents 'coming out', forming pressure groups and attempting to influence policy in ways that were new (Trent, 1994; Jones, 2004). The earliest parents' groups have been dated to the 1930s in the USA (Jones, 2004), but 'were isolated expressions of need' which did not expand beyond the local area (p. 328) – as in the UK it was only after the Second World War that parents' groups gained national policy-influencing momentum.

Rolph notes that in quite practical ways the advent of community-based services, particularly Occupation Centres for children, stimulated contacts between parents which led to their forming social bonds and later local Societies (Rolph, 2002). Certainly there is oral history evidence which testifies to the unimaginable isolation of families with children with learning difficulties prior to the 1950s and even beyond (Rolph *et al.*, 2005). Other historians have cited factors including the growing dominance of psychology which offered an alternative to the medical explanations of mental deficiency, pointing to the importance of environmental factors and the potential for change. However, one should not underestimate the impact of the Second World War. Mathew Thomson has argued that the history of mental deficiency offers some support to those who have argued that welfare state reform emerged out of a gradual process of modernization. The disruption of war offered the chance for voluntary groups and women welfare workers to innovate new mental health services. Furthermore, wartime offered opportunities for individuals who had been labelled 'mentally defective' to take on roles in society, in the armed forces and elsewhere, which were a practical challenge to eugenic pessimism (Gelb, 2004, p. 317). It would be fair to see a constellation of factors contributing to a significant shift in the discourse around mental deficiency so that by the early 1950s written records begin to reveal an attitude more readily characterised as pity than condemnation or fear (Walmsley, 1995b). The association between mental deficiency and lower social classes was challenged by the 'intense middle class familialism of the postwar years' (Jones, 2004, p. 329). Public figures like Brian (now Lord) Rix, then a well-known stage comic actor (Shennan, 1980) admitted to having a family member with learning difficulties, exploding the myth that developmental disability was the prerogative of 'problem families'.

In practice, as noted above, the takeover by the NHS signalled little change except that parents were no longer expected to contribute financially to the maintenance of their sons and daughters in institutions as they had been hitherto (Walmsley, 1995). Thomson also underlines that eugenic anxieties continued to influence the postwar debate. These included the persistence of mental deficiency institutions; the move from the 'social problem group' to the 'problem family'; and continued stigmatisation and fears surrounding the mentally defective (Thomson, 1998a, pp. 270–93). However, almost immediately after the War ended the cause of those detained in institutions was taken up by a non-specialist campaigning organisation, the National Council for Civil Liberties (NCCL). The emergence of a libertarian outcry over mental deficiency is probably the strongest evidence of a change in the attitudes of the general public. The NCCL exposed exploitation and undue restriction of the liberty of patients within mental deficiency institutions in *50,000 Outside the Law* published in 1950. Stainton has analysed this challenge as based on individualistic human rights ideology, a precursor to the 'citizenship' theme which resurfaced in the 1990s (Stainton, 2000).

Ideas and policy 1954–71

The work of the NCCL, coupled with a growing parents' movement – between 1946 and 1955, 50 local Societies were founded in England – pushed the Government to establish the Royal Commission on the Law

Relating to Mental Illness and Mental Deficiency (1954–57). This was the first time Government had taken a comprehensive look at mental deficiency services since the Wood Report in the 1920s. The Royal Commission took evidence from parents' organisations, as well as experts (Shennan, 1980), and was clearly influenced by the idea of community care. It has rightly been seen as a key document in the development of care in the community.

The underpinning philosophy implicitly rejected eugenics. It argued that community services should be available to those who could benefit from them, and there should be no need for formal 'ascertainment' – 'the whole approach should be a positive one offering help and obtaining the co-operation of the patient and his family' (Royal Commission, 1957, p. 101). Where possible, mentally disordered patients should make use of general services. The main point was that the Royal Commission advocated a shift in emphasis from hospitals to community care – it was not 'in the best interests of patients' that they should live for long periods in large or remote institutions, cut off from the 'normal' world and from mixing with other people (Royal Commission, 1957, p. 207). Services should be an integral part of the general health and welfare services. Hospitals would provide in-patient and out-patient treatment for patients who needed specialist medical treatment or continual nursing attention, but local authorities would be responsible for preventive services and community care. This was to include training centres, Occupation Centres, residential accommodation, hostels and general social help and advice. The Royal Commission noted that this would involve 'a considerable expansion of residential and non-residential community health and welfare services' (Royal Commission, 1957, pp. 17–18).

The 1959 Mental Health Act which followed the Royal Commission did not fundamentally undermine hospital care, but had a broad policy of desegregating the mentally disordered and reintegrating them into the community (Unsworth, 1987, pp. 261–2). Politically, this had a broad appeal, and seemed compatible with the welfare state. It was also attractive to the Conservative Right, which under Thorneycroft had promised economies in public spending, carried forward by Powell, in 1961. However it also created pressures for a privatisation of responsibility for the mentally disordered rather than the creation of new welfare services – according with ideas of self-reliance and the importance of the family – ideas which came to policy fruition in the late 1980s. Mathew Thomson has written that the 1959 Act 'may therefore have reformulated the problem of mental deficiency, but the longer-term problem of how to provide effective care for members of society with mental disabilities continued to be a considerable dilemma for the Welfare State' (Thomson, 1998a, p. 296). The new Act was accompanied by new terminology, 'subnormal' replacing the language of 1913 – mental deficiency, feeble-mindedness, idiocy and imbecility. This was the first of the linguistic shifts which have been a prominent feature of the landscape and have arguably consumed a disproportionate share of intellectual energy (Sinason, 1992; Marks, 1999).

Changing ideas about care in the community were reflected in the Seebohm Report (1968). The Seebohm Committee was established in 1965 to consider how health and welfare services should be organised, and to see if a family service was possible. The Committee noted that most patients could live with their families or in hostels if they had adequate medical supervision, through out-patient departments and general practitioners. It also noted that 'much social support is also required for patients, ex-patients and their families to help them directly and to create the most advantageous social environment ... this is what is meant by the community caring' (DHSS, 1968, p. 107). What was termed 'community care' had come to mean treatment and care outside hospitals and residential homes, and it tended to be associated solely with local authority services. However the Seebohm Committee saw these limitations as unfortunate, as such institutions were part of the community, and in the mental health field in particular, it was absurd to ignore the contribution of outpatient departments, day hospitals, general practitioners and nurses (DHSS, 1968, p. 107).

Community care: a changing ideology

Our detailed reading of history has demonstrated that community care existed alongside institutional care (Thomson, 1998a; Walmsley *et al.*, 1999; Walmsley and Rolph, 2001) and was intended to exert a controlling function where, for whatever reason, institutional care was not used. The way the term 'care in the community' was deployed in the 1950s and 1960s suggests that the concept was not systematically defined, its very meaning ambiguous. In 1959, for example, Richard Titmuss, Professor of Social Administration at the London School of Economics, noted that changing ideas represented a move against the bad institution; no such move could be detected against the 'good' institution (Titmuss, 1959, p. 11). In 1961, Titmuss argued at the annual conference of the National Association for Mental Health (NAMH) that the phrase 'community care' conjured up 'a sense of warmth and human kindness, essentially personal and comforting'; he described community care as 'the ever lasting cottage-garden trailer' (Titmuss, 1961, p. 354). Community care has been subject to a number of different meanings in the period under discussion.

Charles Webster has pertinently observed that 'because each new administration has adopted the idea as if it was its own discovery, introducing changes of meaning to suit the prevailing ideology, the extent of the longer term preoccupation with community care tends to be obscured' (Webster, 1996, p. 109). Looking backwards, the sociologist Michael Bayley argued in 1973 that at the time of the *Health and Welfare* White Paper (1963), the Government was thinking entirely in administrative terms, of services in the community. He questioned how 'community' was being defined and argued that by the time of the 1971 White Paper, welfare through the community was not separate to the social services but inextricably interwoven with it. Bayley concluded from his Sheffield case-study that 'care in, by, as part of, and in co-operation with the community can develop most fruitfully if it is linked with the insights of community development' (Bayley, 1973, pp. 342–4). In short, local authority provision was not enough. Thus in the 1960s, community care was defined almost as much as by what it was not – care in long-stay institutions – as by what it was.

The contribution of research

A vigorous strand of research contributed both to the supremacy of community care as a preferred policy option and its manifestations in policy and practice. It is perhaps an irony that community care as a humanitarian alternative to institutional care emerged at a time when 'mental deficiency' had become an academic and policy backwater. In the first third of the twentieth century it had attracted much attention due to its association with what were perceived as pressing social problems. As the perceived danger receded, or became associated with other groups in society, so its importance diminished. Writing in 1958, Alan Clarke and Ann Clarke suggested that the fact that there was no 'cure' for mental deficiency had rendered it unattractive to therapists and research workers (Clarke and Clarke, 1974, p. xiii). Nevertheless research did contribute to changing ideologies of community care. It discredited the existing system of care; demonstrated the potential of alternatives forms of care provision; and demolished the idea of the institution as a therapeutic environment.

Discrediting the existing system

In England, the work of Jack Tizard (1919–79), Neil O'Connor (1917–97) and the Clarkes dominated a number of studies concerning the potential of mental defectives, and the higher than expected IQ levels to be found among inmates of mental handicap hospitals, which discredited the system then in place. It has been suggested that this work 'transformed public attitudes towards mental deficiency and facilitated the humane education and employment of the mentally handicapped'.[2] A number of studies exposed the limitations of current systems of classification, all showing that there were many people in mental handicap hospitals who, on IQ grounds alone, should not be there.

In 1954 Neil O'Connor and Jack Tizard, then based at the Medical Research Council Unit for Research in Occupational Adaptation, later the Social Psychiatry Unit, published the results of a survey of patients in mental deficiency institutions in London, Kent and Surrey. The population from which the five per cent sample was drawn consisted of approximately 11,850 patients, nearly a quarter of the total in England and Wales. Half the patients had been classified as feeble-minded, 5 per cent as idiots and 40 per cent as imbeciles (with an IQ between 25 and 50). But the main finding was that the average IQ of young adult feeble-minded defectives was above 70, suggesting that half the adults classified as feeble-minded in mental deficiency institutions had IQs of over 70. Half the patients did not need any special nursing or supervision; another 24 per cent, while needing no special nursing, were thought to be in need of close supervision (O'Connor and Tizard, 1954, p. 18).

Similarly in 1960, M. W. G. Brandon, a Clinical Psychologist based at the Fountain Hospital in London, reported the results of attempts to assess the abilities and status of 200 adult women classified as feeble-minded. He found that the average IQ of 183 women tested was 81; only 11 per cent had an IQ below 70. Large numbers had physical handicaps, were themselves illegitimate, had lost their parents or had mentally disturbed parents. When the cause of certification was investigated, 25 per cent had been certified mainly because of their having an illegitimate child, and the lack of anyone to take responsibility for them in their late teens and early twenties was also a factor. Brandon investigated whether the original certification of the 200 women and their subsequent years in institutions had been beneficial or necessary, and if not, how this could have been avoided. He concluded 'the majority of those classified as "feeble-minded" in the past, and whose difficulties are in effect more social than intellectual, can be successfully re-established in the community' (Brandon, 1960, pp. 368–9).

Michael Craft, Medical Superintendent at the Oakwood Park Hospital in Conway, reported on the discharge of patients classified as imbeciles from the Royal Western Counties Hospital in the period 1946–55. Of

53 patients, 40 (75 per cent) were working; 9 (17 per cent) were unemployed and on assistance; 16 (30 per cent) had work which had been unchanged since discharge; 10 (19 per cent) had different jobs but were in continuous employment and 27 (51 per cent) had had periods of unemployment requiring assistance. Craft argued that 'this survey of successfully discharged imbeciles emphasised the degree of improvement that deprived individuals may make, but also some remarkable successes with those who although remaining at imbecile level, found a niche which satisfied all' (Craft, 1962, pp. 26–7). J. H. F. Castell, Lecturer in Social Psychology at University College, Swansea, and Peter Mittler, Lecturer in Psychology at Birkbeck College, London, published the results of a survey of admissions to subnormality hospitals in 1961, after the passing of the 1959 Act. They found that the categories of severe subnormality and subnormality introduced by the Act were being applied to patients whose intelligence level did not warrant such classification. Castell and Mittler argued that the category of severe subnormality 'with its implications of very low intelligence, poor response to training, inability to lead an independent life or to guard against exploitation, is apparently being applied to patients whose intelligence level and capacity to respond to suitable training suggest a more favourable prognosis' (Castell and Mittler, 1965, pp. 219–25; Mittler, 1966, p. 21). Together, these studies pointed to considerable failings in the admissions practices of institutions, though they did not point clearly to alternative forms of provision.

Studies of potential

The potential of training and rehabilitation was the focus of a further set of studies. Although there had been interest in the 1920s in the extent to which the feeble-minded could become self-supporting (Lapage, 1911; Fox, 1929), earlier studies had generally been dismissive. Thus in 1929, Dr E. O. Lewis, Medical Investigator to the Wood Committee, had written that:

> imbeciles are incapable not only of earning an independent livelihood, but of contributing materially to their own support. The best that can be expected of imbeciles will be the simplest of routine tasks under supervision. The brightest can manage, in a somewhat irregular fashion, such menial tasks as sweeping, dusting, scrubbing floors, washing earthen-ware and unbreakable articles, and even rough laundry work; here, however, they would need almost

continuous supervision ... In wood-work the best of the imbecile youths can manage rough polishing, sand-papering and hammering large nails, and in needle-work the best of the girls can manage coarse stitching and tacking; few will be able to thread their own needles ... tying shoe laces remains entirely beyond their powers (Clarke and Hermelin, 1955, p. 337).

This view was echoed by A. F. Tredgold as late as 1952:

as a result of training, a considerable proportion can be employed in such simple duties as sweeping and scrubbing floors, polishing brasses, weeding garden paths, collecting potatoes, helping in the laundry, and so on. But they can only do these things under supervision ... None of them can contribute appreciably towards the cost of their upkeep (Clarke and Hermelin, 1955, p. 337).

The research set out to disprove this negative view. This was undertaken mainly by the Medical Research Council Unit. In 1952, Tizard and O'Connor criticised existing training methods in hospitals as being irrelevant to outside employment and as seriously underestimating the potential of trainees. They argued that a large proportion of adults should be regarded as young 'trainable' adults who might eventually be discharged. Although the number of patients on daily and resident licence had increased considerably, much of the training was designed to pass the time rather than produce work of value to the community; the work done in institution workshops bore little relation to the types of work defectives did when on licence; equipment used in workshops was obsolete; little contact was made with commercial firms; there were few incentives, including pay; and supervision was often inadequate. They again drew attention to the high average IQs of trainees as measured by standard intelligence tests; many were merely educationally retarded and could read simple material. Overall they concluded that institutional policy had not been to return defectives to the community but to segregate them (Tizard and O'Connor, 1952, pp. 620–3).

The Clarkes, after challenging the supposition of permanent defect as measured by IQ tests, set up a series of experiments to examine the learning potential of 'ineducable' imbeciles and idiots. They challenged the idea of a rigidly constant IQ. Intellectual retardation was thus not necessarily a permanent and irreversible condition (Clarke and Clarke, 1953, pp. 877–9). In 1955, Alan Clarke and Fliess Hermelin published a study of the 'trainability' of imbeciles which suggested that 'imbeciles' could work reliably and well, earning money, and enjoying their more active work. They concluded 'it seems that the limits to the trainability of imbeciles are very much higher than have been accepted traditionally either in theory or in practice'. Clarke and Hermelin argued that low IQ should not be an excuse for inactivity, but a starting point for planned training and treatment. Similarly qualities such as manual dexterity and motor coordination were not static, but 'capable of improvement within limits which are often ill understood and ill defined' (Clarke and Hermelin, 1955, pp. 337–9).

In 1956, O'Connor and Tizard showed that the traditional view of adult imbeciles as being unable to carry out anything but the simplest tasks was mistaken, and that, provided the right learning experiences were provided, patients with very limited intelligence could sometimes be taught to perform useful work and satisfy the requirements of an industrial contractor. They pointed out that although 21,537 of those deemed to be imbeciles and idiots were suitable for home training, few local authorities provided Occupation Centres, and only 12,658 were receiving training at the end of 1954. There were great differences in the rates of ascertainment in the different parts of England and Wales. They wrote that the 'gross overcrowding and barrack-like austerity of most mental-deficiency hospitals' was an effective way of keeping down the size of waiting lists, along with the lack of Occupation Centres and sheltered workshops, and argued that the basis for an adequate service must be laid in the community (O'Connor and Tizard, 1956, p. 165; Mittler, 1966, p. 20).

Tizard and Jacqueline Grad reported in 1961 on a 1954 survey of the problems experienced by families. They found a shortage of social workers and a lack of liaison between the community and institutional services. Most areas did not have enough Occupation Centres; they were usually in unsatisfactory premises (such as church halls); and the pay and conditions of staff were also poor. However, they did not go so far as to challenge the concept of institutional care, rather advocating a more effective hospital service, closely associated with community-based activity and support. Units for adults and children should be small, located in local communities, with easy admission, discharge and visiting, and with hostels and workshops situated close to one another; the general public would in this way become more accustomed to the 'handicapped' (Tizard and Grad, 1961, p. 131).

Overall, the research described here contributed to confidence in people's ability to respond to training and fulfil useful tasks in industrial employment. These ideas, however, did not point explicitly to the demise of long-stay hospitals, or to the future direction of community care, other than arguing for more of an emphasis on work. While the researchers of the 1950s had shown that people with learning difficulties could learn social and industrial skills, the 1960s were marked more by debate on the *desirability* of rehabilitation, a joint approach to care, and the appropriate training to be carried out, than for any real changes in the pattern of direct care provision (Malin *et al.*, 1980, pp. 54–6).

Debates about the form of community provision

The third major way in which research contributed to ideas about community care was in indicating different approaches to care provision. The most vivid demonstration of how changes to a richer, more stimulating environment could produce substantial improvements in social maturity and verbal intelligence was the 'Brooklands' experiment, carried out under the supervision of Jack Tizard. In an early report (1960), he put forward some very practical arguments for moving away from reliance on long-stay hospitals. He noted that the number of severely subnormal children who survived infancy had shown a striking increase, but that the number of children who went into mental deficiency hospitals was restricted by the number of beds available, and the pressure to find more places was bound to grow. He also argued that few attempts had been made in the previous 30 years to think through the basis for institutional care and to see what changes were desirable to bring it into line with changing mental health needs, and increased understanding of them (Tizard, 1960, p. 1041).

Tizard's project was funded by the NSMHCA, a notable instance of the way parents' groups exerted influence on research to influence policy direction. He took a group of 32 severely subnormal children from a large and overcrowded hospital in London and arranged for them to be looked after in a small, family-type unit, in Reigate, Surrey, run as far as possible as a normal pre-school nursery. A control group, matched for sex, age, type of defect and IQ remained in the hospital. The Brooklands children were educated according to their mental age, using modified nursery and infant school methods. Tizard found that this had a dramatic effect on the children, writing that 'they are energetic and full of fun. They are for the most part docile and easy to manage; and they are fond of the staff and the staff of them. If the contrast sounds too good to be true it is because the change itself has exceeded our expectations' (Tizard, 1960, p. 1044). After one year, the children had increased by eight months in mental age as measured by a verbal intelligence test, as against three months for the controls; while in personal independence they had increased six months as against three months for the controls. Tizard argued that the role of the large hospital should be examined anew; a different type of educational programme would meet the needs of the children more effectively and the psychological development of handicapped children could be modified by changes in their management (Tizard, 1960, pp. 1044–5; Mittler, 1966, pp. 22–3).

In *Community Services for the Mentally Handicapped* (1964), Tizard reported on the Brooklands experiment and made a broader series of recommendations. He argued that large institutions tended to be remote from the centres of population; they easily became isolated from developments in medicine, psychiatry and education; they wasted specialist services; it was difficult to attract and keep good staff; and visiting was also difficult. Tizard argued that the costs of small units need not be greater than that of larger establishments, if specialist services were pooled (Tizard, 1964, p. 161). He recommended hostels for 'high grade defectives who are working out', and for 'lower grade dependent defectives'. He recognised it was desirable that the hostels should cater for both men and women since their function would be 'to prepare school-leavers and young adults for independent living in ordinary lodgings or their own homes' (Tizard, 1964, p. 174). The residents would normally go out to work in the daytime. But the main need was for long-stay homes for adults. Again, this provision should be in small family-type units, close to sheltered workshops. Part of the argument was that day and residential services should be integrated so that services might be used both by patients living in their own homes and those in residential care. If schools and workshops catered for larger numbers, it might be possible to keep hostels small (Tizard, 1964, pp. 175–6; Jones, 1975, p. 4).

The Brooklands experiment was followed by studies of hospital educational facilities. In 1966, Peter Mittler and Mary Woodward published a survey of 403 children admitted to 17 subnormality hospitals in England and Wales in 1962. Of 155 who could be given standard IQ tests, 98 (24 per cent) had IQs over 50; of these, 57 (14 per cent of the total sample) had IQs over 70, and 15 (4 per cent) had IQs over 100. Of 100 teaching staff, 22 per cent had the appropriate NAMH qualification; 13 per cent were qualified teachers; but 57 per cent had no qualification. The fact that so many children had IQs over 50 – a range of intelligence within which children were usually considered suitable for education in schools – led Mittler and Woodward to question why they were admitted to subnormality hospitals and whether hospitals were suitable educational establishments; some children who could not remain at home were admitted to hospital because there was no alternative. They supported policies designed to bring the educational work of hospitals under education authorities (Mittler and Woodward, 1966, pp. 16–25; Mittler, 1966, p. 24).

There was debate about other types of community provision, such as hostels. Hostels had begun to be developed tentatively in the 1930s, and had been expanded for groups of evacuated children during the Second World War. F. J. S. Esher, a Consultant Psychiatrist, argued in 1965 that there should be two types of hostels for the subnormal – 'custodial hostels' for patients who needed life-long care, and 'rehabilitatory hostels', to act as a half-way house between the hospital and the outside world. Custodial hostels could be regarded as a modern replacement for institutional care, for patients to enjoy some measure of freedom in the community. All patients should go out to work during the day, and visits to relatives at weekends should be encouraged. 'Rehabilitatory' hostels should not be sited in hospital grounds, and should be between 12 and 20 places. The aim should be to make patients self sufficient. Esher aimed to provide a clearer concept of the local authority role in providing residential care for subnormal patients, that of 'homely care' (Esher, 1965, pp. 124–5). Similarly Peter Mittler concluded in 1966 that 'hostels of various kinds should be more widely available, both to avoid the admission of new patients, and to facilitate the discharge and rehabilitation of long-stay hospital patients' (Mittler, 1966, p. 27). At the Wessex Regional Hospital Board (RHB), Albert Kushlick suggested the need for research into methods of management in long-term hospitals and the training of personnel. It was important that anti-therapeutic hospital routines were not continued in new or upgraded facilities (Kushlick, 1969, p. 1197).

This body of research began to give shape to the type of community provision that could develop alongside hospital care. One of the best known innovations of the 1960s was the Slough experiment, run by the NSMHCA (Mittler and Castell, 1964, p. 873; Baranyay, 1971). This instituted a hostel associated with an Occupation Centre within walking distance for young adults of both sexes. The hostel was run by 'houseparents' a husband and wife couple, and became an influential model for community provision.[3]

Overall, there were important advances in the understanding of what by the early 1970s was termed 'mental retardation'; by 1974 the Clarkes found it necessary to restructure and rewrite their textbook and extend the coverage from 18 to 25 chapters (Clarke and Clarke, 1974, p. xix). However none of the research fundamentally challenged institutional care as the dominant service model. Rather it argued for reform and development of community provision as a positive adjunct. It took sociologists to put forward arguments which fundamentally challenged institutions as a form of care.

Sociologists and critiques of institutional life

The literature on classification and rehabilitation had been dominated by psychologists. Towards the end of the period, however, sociologists began to make an impact, particularly through a critique of institutions. The most influential publication was Erving Goffman's collection of essays entitled *Asylums*, first published in the USA in 1961 and in Great Britain two years later. It was Goffman who developed the concept of the 'total institution', of which the enclosed mental hospital was in many ways the exemplar. In total institutions, people assumed the status of patient and became incorporated in the management of what was deemed to be deviant behaviour; it involved rituals of degradation, segregation from normal life and the imposition of a new and damaged identity which reshaped the reactions of others to the victim of this process, now relegated to a morally inferior social position (Martin, 1984, pp. 31–2). Goffman was later to write that entry into institutional care entailed what he called 'curtailment of the self' – the individual cast off one set of roles (mother, daughter, husband, wife) and took on another (resident, patient, inmate). Goffman was thus an early and influential exponent of labelling theory, which other American sociologists had built up with particular reference to delinquency.

Goffman was not alone in this thinking. Almost simultaneously, in a book published in 1961, Russell Barton, Physician Superintendent of Severalls Hospital, and Consultant Psychiatrist for Essex County Council, wrote of the 'institutional mind and the subnormal mind'. Following Goffman, he argued that the characteristic authority evolved in institutions had three distinctive elements – authority was of the echelon kind; it was reflected in matters of dress, deportment, social intercourse, manners and so on; and misbehaviours in one sphere of life were held against people's standing in other spheres. Barton wrote that the inmate 'cannot easily escape from the press of judgemental officials and from the enveloping tissue of constraint'. The effect was 'a production of a pattern of culture – attitudes, behaviour and values – so different from the pattern of culture in the rest of the community that adaptation to life outside the institution requires considerable and difficult readjustment'. Barton listed what he termed 'seven deadly sins' of institutions – loss of contact with the outside world; enforced idleness; bossiness of medical and nursing staff; loss of personal friends, possessions and personal events; excessive use of drugs; a bad ward atmosphere; and loss of prospects outside the institution. Particularly difficult was loss of personal possessions – 'even today, many patients have no locker on which they could be encouraged to put photographs, no wardrobe in which to hang their frocks and suits, no chest of drawers in which to keep their clothes' (Barton, 1961, pp. 37–44).

Social science research was also a source of ideas about the direction of community care. Peter Townsend and Richard Titmuss were directly involved with research on the personal social services; with political groups such as the Fabian Society; and with the training of social workers. Research that they supervised and conducted was crucial in exposing the slow progress in implementing care in the community. Moreover they also illustrated ambiguities in the vocabulary and basic concepts. Peter Townsend's study *The Last Refuge* (1962), an ethnographic study of residential homes for older people, was influential in Britain. Townsend was concerned with the relationship between the size of the institution and the quality of care that was provided. He showed that smaller homes had small staffs, with less specialisation of labour; relationships between the staff and the residents were closer and more informal; and the customs and practices of home and community life were more closely simulated (Tizard, 1964, p. 157). Townsend's arguments pointed to hostels as small and inexpensive, alongside sheltered workshops – the Slough model.

In the late 1960s, Townsend's critique was boosted by Pauline Morris's study *Put Away* (1969), based on a large-scale survey of 35 subnormality hospitals in England and Wales and financed by the NSMHCA. In the foreword, Townsend wrote that the accumulating evidence of social influences on intelligence had weakened if not destroyed the eugenic case for social segregation; there were serious doubts about the hospital being the right environment for the care of the subnormal; and most might be better cared-for in sheltered family or community care than in hospitals or hostels. Morris had shown that 61 per cent of patients were in hospital complexes of more than 1000 beds each, and only 1 per cent were in single rooms – 38 per cent were in wards with 60 beds or more (Townsend, 1969, p. xxiv).

Morris stressed that patients were for the most part looked after by people who cared, and many accepted 'those whom society chooses to reject' (Morris, 1969, pp. 314–15; Jones, 1975, pp. 9–11). But she provided a devastating picture of conditions in the larger institutions. She found that in many institutions, the stock of clothing was communal, meaning that after laundry it was not returned to individuals. Hospitals did not provide many items of clothing, and most were 'dull, unimaginative and often ill-fitting'. Often the clothes that were worn were poorly matched, 'nondescript and baggy' (Morris, 1969, pp. 95–7). Morris showed that although the smaller homes seemed more comfortable and less regimented, the psychological implications of subnormality were neglected, and in this respect the smaller homes were more isolated from theories of rehabilitation than the larger institutions (Morris, 1969, p. 276). A high proportion of patients lived in buildings that were dilapidated and decrepit, two-thirds of which had been built before 1900. Most were geographically remote. Although it was assumed that patients required skilled medical and nursing care, over 80 per cent were able to walk, and the amount of serious physical or mental illness among them was small. There seemed to be little consensus about treatment objectives. Morris recommended that the existing hospitals should provide accommodation and treatment for those who required constant medical and nursing care. They should become Day Centres providing outpatient medical and psychiatric treatment for the majority of people who would live in hostels (Morris, 1969, pp. 309–15).

Following the publication of Robb's *Sans Everything* (1967), another exposé of unacceptable conditions, the Ministry of Health knew that abuses in hospitals needed to be confronted. The trigger for action came in July 1967 when the *News of the World* newspaper received from a former employee of Ely Hospital, a subnormality hospital near Cardiff, allegations of ill-treatment and stealing by members of staff; indifference on the part of the chief male nurse to complaints; and lack of care by the Physician Superintendent, and another doctor. A detailed enquiry was carried out by a Committee under the chairmanship of Geoffrey Howe, QC. The report, a model of its kind, concluded that 'the situation at Ely has proved to be sufficiently disturbing to make [the complainant's] concern well justified' (Jones, 1975, pp. 6–9; Martin, 1984, p. 29; Webster, 2002, pp. 118–21). Far-reaching changes were recommended in almost every aspect of the hospital's activities. One aspect that was emphasised was the need for closer liaison with the local authority and for some development of community-based services.

Richard Crossman, as Secretary of State for Social Services, inherited the report. He insisted on the publication of the whole report and set up a Working Party which met for two years and made sweeping proposals for improvement. Members included Peter Townsend, Pauline Morris and Geoffrey Howe. A number of interim measures were taken, including (in 1969) the setting up of the Hospital Advisory Service (Jones, 1975, pp. 6–11). Crossman's biographer writes that he transformed a potential administrative disaster for the Department of Health and Social Security (DHSS) into the occasion for putting the spotlight on what until then had been a shamefully neglected area of the NHS (Crossman, 1977; Howard, 1990, 1991 edn., pp. 294–5). Thus the powerful sociological critique of institutional care had by the late 1960s been augmented by evidence of scandals relating to ill-treatment, stealing, and indifference on the part of staff.

Conclusion

This chapter has explored the ideas behind community care in the period 1948–71. It has traced the evolution of thinking about how to care for and manage people with learning difficulties over the twentieth century, from the eugenic approaches characteristic of the early twentieth century through to challenges to institutions as the preferred model of care in the 1950s and 1960s. It has shown that there was a broad shift from control to care in the period, and that there was a discernible point around mid-century when changing ideas making community options more acceptable than in the prewar period, and more directed towards the improvement of individuals' life experiences and opportunities, began to surface. We have stressed the significance of the creation of parents' groups, and their success in demonstrating that any family, not just those in the lower social classes, could find themselves with a child with learning difficulties, and discussed the impact of research, often funded by voluntary organisations, alongside the influence of scandals, such as Ely Hospital. Social psychology research had discredited the existing system of care by illustrating the flawed system of classification, highlighting the potential for training and rehabilitation to make a difference and demolishing the idea of the institution as a therapeutic environment. Having explored the ideas behind care in the community in this period, Chapter 3 will trace how they were embodied in structures and organisations and assess the extent to which a policy of care in the community was implemented in the period 1948–71. It will move from what was said to what was done, or not done.

Notes

1. Bedfordshire Record Office, Bedford: Beds He sub m 6/1 1949.
2. *Guardian*, October 1997.
3. Luton Mencap Society, *Yearbook 1967* (Luton, 1968).

2
Ideology, Ideas and Care in the Community, 1971–2001

Jan Walmsley

Introduction

In this chapter we examine the interrelationship between ideas about community care which informed broad policy development, and some very specific learning disability ideologies and developments which have given it its particular flavour in the second part of our period. Learning disability policy has much in common with the direction of travel in the wider health and social care context, but it has developed a distinctive rhetoric which, we argue, is attributable to its ideological history. Ideas which have come from the disability movement, with which learning disability has increasingly been associated, have become highly influential in informing policy development. Citizenship and independent living supported by Direct Payments have been ideals espoused by the disabled people's movement which have percolated into the broader policy arena. Organisations, known as 'self-advocacy groups', which represent people with learning difficulties, sprang up from the 1980s, a development possibly unique to this period, and one which paralleled the growth of 'user' groups across the spectrum of people who use community care services. In some respects the ideas and idealism of activists have been made to serve the baser interests of politicians to cut costs and reduce dependence on welfare agencies.

Ideals might push policy in a particular direction – *Valuing People* and its companion White Papers in Wales and Scotland are highly idealistic in their aspirations for choice, independence, rights and inclusion, and it is possible to trace the influences which pushed policy in this direction. Equally, as Morris (2004) cogently pointed out, although the policies are in place, practice lags behind, for a wide raft of reasons, some of which will be illustrated in Part IV. For example, although it is apparent that the service users whose lives are described in Chapter 10 have experienced a richer life as policy has changed, there are definite restrictions on the degree to which any of the three can be said to have reached the sort of life envisioned in *Valuing People*.

Community care: from place to market

In the earlier period of our book, relocating people with learning difficulties from large institutions to smaller (but still sizable) hostels in towns and cities, along with the establishment of Day Centres for children, and later adults, was seen as community care. Essentially this is a concept in which bricks and mortar are the salient things to change. Means *et al.* (2003) argue that, by the 1970s, community care was shifting to exclude residential care of the hostel type, to free up resource to use on non-institutional provision such as home and day care. In discussing the historical social geography of 'mental retardation' in the USA, Deborah Metzel notes that it was at this time, in the 1970s, that this relocation became a 'volatile issue' of public concern as homes were mooted in residential areas (2004, p. 433).

The move away from a bricks and mortar conception of community care developed further in the late 1980s as governments began to recognise the significance of family (informal) care and the need to support informal carers. Community care became more explicitly associated with supporting family and home-based care. The White Paper *Growing Older* (1981) noted that '... the primary sources of support and care for elderly people are informal and voluntary ... . Care *in* the community must increasingly mean *by* the community' (DOH, 1981, p. 3). It was families that were seen as the principal sources of support and care, and the role of public services was an enabling one. A subsequent White Paper *Caring for People* (1989) acknowledged that the great bulk of community care was provided by friends, family and neighbours, and community care was no longer seen as the prerogative of public services; the voluntary and private sectors were equally important (DOH, 1989, p. 13). At this point a distinct rhetoric of promoting independence is discernible in policy pronouncements: 'providing the right level of intervention and support to enable people to achieve maximum independence and control over their own lives' (DOH, 1989, para. 2.2).

It is here that the idea of community services supporting citizenship becomes more pronounced. This may be regarded as a triumph for the sorts of ideas discussed later in the chapter, but such a conception of care in the community was also seen as an alternative to expensive involvement by the social services and by the then Conservative Government as a cost-cutting service (Digby, 1989, p. 93). Andrew Scull has written extensively on the reasons for the triumph of community-based over institutional solutions, and argues powerfully that community care ideals 'allowed governments to save money while simultaneously giving their policy a humanitarian gloss' (Scull, 1984, p. 139). It was because the plans promised major cost savings that they drew extensive support from right-wing political figures. He writes that 'the primary value of that rhetoric (though far from its authors' intent) seems to have been its usefulness as ideological camouflage, allowing economy to masquerade as benevolence and neglect as tolerance' (Scull, 1984, pp. 152–3). In the later 1990s, and the early twenty-first-century, with the advent of Direct Payments-individualised funding, we see an even further shift away from buildings, to individualised conceptions where the user as consumer becomes the driver of the types of services s/he receives. Although used by only a minority in practice, in the minds of policy makers this is the way forward (DOH, 2005). At this point, the term 'community care' appears to lose its currency, to be replaced by 'social care'.

Community care was also seen in terms of relationships, less by policy makers than by academics. In 1973 Michael Bayley was perhaps the first to draw the distinction between care *in* the community and care *by* the community. The importance of social relationships in enabling people with learning difficulties to participate fully in society was an important theme of commentators associated with normalisation and integration, with ideas associated with citizen advocacy and staff roles as a stepping stone to 'valued social relationships' being important messages (King's Fund Centre, 1988). Community care as essentially being about relationships was subsequently elaborated by Martin Bulmer who in 1987 stated ' "community care" is concerned with the resources available outside formal institutional structures, particularly in the informal relationships of the family, friends and neighbours as a means of providing care' (p. 45). It is this association with relationships that has been distinctively, though not exclusively, linked to learning disability. It may be that this important link has been threatened if not lost as community care becomes ever more individualised via individualised payments and an emphasis on people as 'citizens' with all the ramifications of autonomy that go with the concept (Burton and Kagan, 2006). Community care can also, as feminists of the 1980s and early 1990s were keen to point out, mean care by families, particularly women (Graham, 1983). This is without doubt the most enduring form of community care, not an invention of the late twentieth century, but lasting from at least the eighteenth century (Walmsley and Rolph, 2001), and remaining the mainstay of people's support well into the twenty-first century. Mencap estimated that in 2005, 29,000 people still lived at home with parents over 70 (*Viewpoint*, 2005, p. 18).

From about 1990, community care became a shorthand for the introduction of the market, competing providers from the private and voluntary sector joining with statutory services as care providers, with major ramifications for the ways services are delivered, and for the economic basis of care, which changed from being a social good in the 1970s to a market commodity in the last decade of the twentieth century. We show in Part IV how rapidly in England at least, this prolif-eration of providers developed so that community care became an often bewildering array of provision, much still in buildings – residential care, Day Centres – but largely comprising a web of provision built around more flexible people resources, such as support workers, home carers, and carers allowances and similar, to ensure that the valuable work of informal/family carers continues and people's independence is supported. It should be noted that between 1971 and 2001, legislation intended for all dependent groups became the norm in England. People with learning difficulties were included in ideological shifts in the meaning of community care which were intended as applicable across the board. However, learning disability retained a distinct identity, as exemplified in *Valuing People*. In the rest of this chapter the distinctive role of learning disability specific ideas, particularly normalisation, is explored.

Sociological critiques of institutions

The most powerful and influential ideologies informing campaigns for policy change across the board in this era appear to have been sociologi-cal critiques of institutions. These critiques, as noted in the previous chapter, addressed the whole range of client groups – older people, people with physical disabilities as well as people with learning difficulties. Townsend's *The Last Refuge* (1962) (relating to old people's homes), Robb's *Sans Everything* (1967), Pauline Morris's *Put Away* (1969) and Maureen Oswin's *The Empty Hours* (1971) all painted a bleak picture of isola-tion, meaningless routines, impoverished surroundings and demoralised residents. Morris demonstrated that most residents were there, not because of intellectual limitations, but for social reasons, and lack of

alternatives, thus laying the conceptual groundwork for policy change.
Goffman's four characteristics of institutional living – rigidity of routine,
block treatment, depersonalisation and social distance (as explained in
Asylums 1961) – began to be used explicitly by some researchers as a way
of measuring quality of provision. Norma Raynes and Roy King created
scales directly from these four characteristics in order to study 16 environments housing children. Their finding, that hospital settings tended
to an institutional orientation while hostels tended to what they called an
'inmate orientation', should not come as a surprise (Raynes and King,
1972). What is notable is the attempt to translate Goffman's abstractions
into a practical rating scale.

The fact that policy moved against institutional care after 1971 is not
explained by the critiques – but they did pave the way for the new direction of policy, as did normalisation and social role valorisation (SRV),
probably the most decisive influences on late twentieth-century services
and thinking about learning disability.

Normalisation

Normalisation ideologies arose in Scandinavia at the very end of the
1950s (Bank-Mikkelson, 1969). Normalisation ideas espoused by Nirje
(1969, 1970) and Bank-Mikkelson (1980) in Scandinavia brought with
them the discourse of ordinary living. The Scandinavian version of
normalisation aimed at creating 'an existence for the mentally retarded
as close to normal living conditions as possible ... making normal,
mentally retarded people's housing, education, working and leisure
conditions' (Bank-Mikkelson, 1980, p. 56). In practice this meant challenging institutional segregation as a matter of right, although Emerson
(1992) contends that this was compatible with segregated settings, not
requiring integration to be successful. Thus, changes might include
living, working and taking pleasure in different places, just as happens
in ordinary life.

Specific practice-related ramifications of this version of normalisation
included such innovations as the Brooklands, Wessex and Slough experiments. The Wessex initiative was the brainchild of Albert Kushlick and
entailed creating 'two living units of 20–25 places designed to provide
for all residential care needs for all of the mentally handicapped children from a total population of 100,000' (Kushlick, 1974, p. 309). They
were situated in towns, though administered from the local hospitals
Coldeast and Tatchbury Mount. The children attended Junior Training
Centres (JTCs) (if acceptable to the managers thereof) and had most

medical needs provided by general practitioners (GPs). The fact that at the time this relatively modest experiment was seen as somewhat daring is an interesting commentary upon the conceptual framework which dominated thinking at the time. Hospital care was increasingly discredited, but its total replacement remained unthinkable.

Social role valorisation

SRV elaborated on normalisation and is closely associated with Wolf Wolfensberger, a US-based academic. Wolfensberger's SRV argued for: 'the utilisation of means which are as culturally normative as possible, in order to establish and/or maintain personal behaviours and characteristics which are as culturally normative as possible' (1972, p. 28). The renaming SRV was intended to emphasise enhancing people's behaviour, appearances, experiences, status and reputation so that they would not be socially devalued. Wolfensberger built on Erving Goffman's work. Not only did Goffman critique hospital living in *Asylums*, he also offered in *Stigma* (1963) an explanation for social devaluation. Stigma, he argued, is the product of social interactions. It is not the stigmatising condition in itself which creates the difficulties for individuals, rather the way people respond to it. Thus SRV, by offering people 'valued social roles', was believed to be a route to reversing stigma by improving societal perceptions of people with learning disabilities. The ramifications were quite extensive. Association with other devalued individuals was to be discouraged. Special services, reserved for stigmatised groups, should give way to services which cater for all. Caution was to be exercised over social image – men should wear ties and suits, women should be carefully made up with styled hair to increase social acceptance (Wolfensberger, 1983; Wolfensberger and Tullman, 1989). Adult image was all important. There should be avoidance of 'childish' associations – people who liked walking round with a teddy bear should be discouraged (Brechin and Walmsley, 1989). We can see how this influenced the lives of people with learning difficulties described in Part IV.

Although normalisation/SRV has been criticised for placing the onus on individuals to change, as illustrated in Chapter 14, there was acknowledgement that efforts needed to be made on the side of society. Citizen advocacy encouraged 'valued' citizens to reach out to devalued individuals and offer them a place in their networks, as well as assistance in speaking up for their rights. This injunction extended also to staff who were encouraged to extend normal professional boundaries and include people in their own worlds outside work (King's Fund Centre, 1988).

We see an example of this in practice in relation to Yvette who was supported by staff for years after she was formally their responsibility (Chapter 10). Communities were encouraged to be welcoming, with a especial emphasis on churches as a nodal point for community inclusion. In particular, services and service providers were seen as key agents in the promotion of 'an ordinary life' (Williams and Atkinson, 1989). Although this was rarely very effective, Yvette's life story shows that occasionally it does work and how important these ties are.

Influence on UK policy

Normalisation and SRV have been remarkably influential in the design and philosophy of learning disability services since the 1970s. The Jay Report was probably the first official report relating to learning disability to speak the language of rights influenced explicitly by SRV. It argued that all people with mental handicap should live in the community with support from the non-medical caring professions. Its key principles were

- mentally handicapped people have a right to enjoy normal patterns of life within the community,
- mentally handicapped people have the right to be treated as individuals and
- mentally handicapped people will require additional help from the communities in which they live and from professional services if they are to develop their maximum potential as individuals.

It recommended the ending of the dual system of hospital and local care and a shift to local care, with a corresponding transfer of resources from the NHS to local authorities (*Report of the Committee of Enquiry*, 1979). The preamble to the All Wales Strategy (AWS) initiated in 1983 also makes clear reference to normalisation (Felce *et al.*, 1998). Walmsley and Johnson (2003) have also identified normalisation/SRV influences in more recent initiatives, such as the promotion of the valued roles of author and researcher for people with learning difficulties.

A striking feature of normalization, at a time when 'spread' of innovation was a policy preoccupation (Oldham, 2004), was the sustained and successful campaign by Wolfensberger's allies in the UK, such as Campaign for Mentally Handicapped (CMH, later Values Into Action), to influence local policy makers and professional groups through PASS and PASSING, workshops which few senior or middle managers in learning disability services avoided in the 1980s. Checklists such as O'Brien and Lyle's well-known *Five Accomplishments* (of services) (1987) offered a straightforward and practical (if simplistic) route map for improvement:

• Physical presence
• Choice
• Competence
• Respect
• Participation

The influential London-based charitable foundation, the King's Fund, adopted and reworked normalisation into a characteristically British formulation, *An Ordinary Life* (King's Fund, 1980), dropping much of the unseemly jargon accompanying Wolfensberger's writings. This further increased its widespread acceptance. With its relatively simple message and lack of self doubt, it can safely be said that few contemporary philosophies have become so quickly or consistently embedded in practice, and careful reading of *Valuing People* discloses some continuing influence, 40 years on, as discussed in more detail in Part IV.

Practice implications

Most of the notable developments in community-based services between 1971 and the late 1990s can be linked to normalisation or SRV. Many were beneficial. Walker and Walker (1998) compared older people's and learning disability services, and found the philosophy of the latter far more conducive to productive living and choice than the former. Celebrated and relatively generously resourced experiments such as the Cardiff NIMROD project (Blunden, 1980) or the Bristol Wells Road service (Ward, 1989) were held up as role models to emulate. The concept of welcoming communities, the acceptance that, however difficult, as they left hospital people should be placed near their families and local ties, the emphasis on getting real jobs rather than live life in sheltered workshops all were linked to these ideas (Williams and Atkinson, 1989). If association with 'valued' citizens was to be achieved, then large group activities were to be avoided. Small size living units housing small groups of people (group homes) were advocated. SRV gave staff a key role in reversing societal attitudes. The practice, so widespread in the early decades of community care, of infantilising people with learning difficulties was discouraged. Integration, meaning the use of local facilities rather than specialist services in education, health and leisure pursuits was fundamental (Booth *et al.*, 1990). Normalisation/SRV is also associated with the discrediting of large-scale Adult Training Centres (ATCs) in favour of community-based options – work, volunteering and leisure. In more doctrinaire applications the location of services was also an issue. Not only should homes be in 'valued' parts of the town, proximity to cemeteries, slaughterhouses and zoos was seen to promote negative associations with death or with animals and should be avoided at all costs (Wolfensberger and Tullman, 1989).

Some negative consequences can also be discerned. The value of friendships between people with learning difficulties, often a sustaining feature of long-stay institutions for individuals, was discounted (Chappell, 1997). Deinstitutionalisation often severed these links, and SRV had little to say about it. Practice could be doctrinaire and rigid. Dorothy Atkinson has shown how 'institutional' can refer to a style of care that denies individual choice, as much as to the type or size of a building (Atkinson, 1998c, pp. 13–26). Studies by Collins (1992, 1993, 1994) and Sinson (1993) demonstrated that institutional practices, far from being outlawed in the new style living units, were reproduced. Indeed, small homes might have been worse in their isolation, with staff out of touch with new ideas. Stephen Thornton, for example, manager of the so-called Priority Services (mental health, mental handicap and community health) in Cambridge 1983–89, commented: 'I still think we were creating mini institutions, a mindset from hospital to community, and I still fear for those people in those homes, there isn't proper checking, I don't think we got it right in the community'.[1]

Occupation Centres, subsequently renamed ATCs, did not, on the whole, disappear, despite some experiments with alternatives. Instead they were renamed Social Education Centres (SECs), contract work was, by and large, discontinued, and those attending were subject to a life of perpetual leisure and 'education', but education for what was rarely articulated. Some service users disliked the abandonment of 'work' in Day Centres – as one said 'I know how to cook. What use gardening, I haven't got a garden' (cited in Walmsley, 1995b, p. 135), regretting the loss of the associations, however exploitative, with the adult world of wages, regular working hours and productivity. Similarly, families were distrustful of the new ideas, suspecting, often with justification, that the running down of Hospitals and Day Services was a cost-cutting exercise more than anything else (Cox and Pearson, 1995).

Challenges to normalisation/SRV

Normalisation did not go unchallenged. On the one hand, dissent was heard from the parents in 'Rescare' who wanted to protect their children's placements in the institutions (Cox and Pearson, 1995) while trade unions protested vigorously at the implications for jobs in institutions (Oswin, 2000). On the other hand, and from a different standpoint, some feminist sociologists spoke out against what they perceived as the unquestioned dogma of normalisation which could, if unchecked, lead to a desire to 'normalise' people's individual differences and a requirement that they should conform in order to gain acceptance (Chappell, 1992). In particular, it was pointed out that what is 'normal' in a given culture is deeply contested and can too easily be translated into white, middle-class and male (Brown and Smith, 1992). From another standpoint some feminists criticised community care as a movement, arguing that it burdened women carers (Graham, 1983), some going as far as to advocate a reinvention of institutional care so that the 'burden' could be placed firmly back in the hands of the state (Dalley, 1988).

Normalisation's influence on practice, although overall positive in comparison with what went before, has also been criticised. Brown and Walmsley (1997) cite instances of questionable practices, such as discouraging the use of wheelchairs and sign language as negative imagery; failure to acknowledge that some people really do have extraordinary needs; and the devaluing elements of discouraging association between people with learning disabilities in favour of the company of, often indifferent or hostile, 'valued people'. People using 'ordinary' buses or living in 'ordinary' streets may be subject to name calling and harassment. Brown and Walmsley have concluded that 'it is too often interpreted wrongly by front line staff and managers, and can be used as an excuse for not providing training or specialist techniques when they are clearly a requirement' (1997, p. 231). Further critiques, more fundamental in ethos, have emanated from the disability movement, and it is these we turn to next.

The social model of disability

Whilst normalisation/SRV has had far-reaching impact on the shape of learning disability services, not just in the UK, but across the English speaking world (see Part III of this book), one could argue that the social model of disability is one of the most significant influences on the philosophical landscape across the whole of social policy in the late twentieth century. Its influence on thinking in relation to oppressed and excluded groups is profound. As Mike Oliver commented, with reference to Tony Blair's stated determination to remove barriers to people fulfilling their potential, 'we are all social modellists now!' (Oliver, 2004, p. 7).

The social model of disability defines disability as the societal response to impairment. As Tom Shakespeare summed it up 'people are disabled by social barriers and failures of provision, not by their bodies' (Shakespeare, 2003, p. 28). The contrast with more traditional definitions of disability are sharp. Whereas the social model locates problems in society – barriers to full participation by people with a variety of impairments – both traditional, often called medical, and normalisation/SRV models locate the problem in the individual. When it comes to a consideration of its influence on learning disability it is worth noting that Shakespeare specifically refers to 'bodies', not 'brains' or 'minds', in his definition. This is not insignificant – people who write about the social model do not always consider impairments which are located in the brain rather than in the body. As a consequence, our understanding of the barriers people with learning difficulties experience is far less well developed (Chappell, 1997).

It was social model thinking which led to the conceptualisation of independent living as a goal for disabled people, to be achieved by employing appropriate personal assistance (Morris, 1993). This individualised market model has become mainstreamed in social policy thinking (e.g., the 2005 Health and Social Care Green Paper in England) (DOH, 2005) and has made some impact on the way learning disability policy is conceived in *Valuing People* (see Chapter 4). It was, at least in part, campaigning by disabled people which led to legislation that made it mandatory for local authorities to make Direct Payments available so that assistance was under the direct control of disabled people, rather than mediated through Care Managers (Shakespeare, 2003) and which has led to the passage of a series of Acts designed to outlaw discrimination against disabled people. Furthermore, disability activists have rejected the idea that care is what they need, as opposed to obtaining assistance to lead the types of lives they choose as active and equal citizens (Kestenbaum, 1996).

People with learning difficulties have undoubtedly benefited from their policy association with disabled people. They are entitled to Direct Payments and are covered by the Disability Discrimination Act. But it is important to note that bodily impairment is the primary model in disability – adapting Direct Payments to suit people with learning difficulties has been a slow and painful process (Swindon People First, 2002; Race *et al.*, 2005).

There are other differences between the disabled people's movement and the movement to promote the rights of people with learning difficulties. Whilst people with learning difficulties and their allies have been trying to establish the principle of a common humanity, groups representing disabled people have been claiming the right to define and name themselves as a group with a distinctive separate identity (Walmsley, 2002; Clement, 2004). The disability movement has promoted a positive stance towards what some people would term 'segregation', by encouraging peer-support, peer-advocacy, disability arts, disability pride and disability culture. Some advocate separate schools for disabled children. This is a stance in stark contrast to advocates of normalisation.

The self-organisations of disabled people challenge prevailing negative stereotypes. The arts have been used as a means of fighting back against the disabling dominant culture (Campbell and Oliver, 1996; Vasey, 2004). For many, 'coming out' as a self proclaimed disabled person has important political meaning (Wendell, 1996). Liz Crow, for example: 'for years now the social model of disability has enabled me to confront, survive and even surmount countless situations of exclusion and discrimination' (1996, p. 207). A perception that the impairment itself is not the problem, that it lies in societal structures and attitudes, has been tremendously liberating for many disabled people. It has led to the re-adoption of particular terms, such as 'cripple' (Mairs, 1986), to express defiance at the world and has undoubtedly contributed to a radical shift in the way disability, and disabled people, are viewed. The extent to which this radical shift applies to people with learning difficulties is less marked (Walmsley, 2001).

The social model of disability and its relationship to learning disability

Critics of normalisation argue that it was imposed on people with learning disabilities by others (Chappell, 1997). Arguably the social model is equally external to people with learning disabilities. It is hard to locate a discovery of barriers in what are, admittedly, the quite limited writings by people with learning disabilities (an exception being Aspis, 2000).

The use of language is an area where the two groups have differed. The disability movement has insisted on the use of the term 'disabled people' to convey the idea that disability is created by society. However, what has been called People First Language seeks to put the person first and the disability second (Chapman, 2005). In this thinking, people with disabilities are people, first and foremost. Indeed, the People First slogan 'Label Jars, not People' itself emphasises this anti-labelling position. There is an obvious tension in establishing a self-advocacy group on the basis of belonging to the social category 'people with learning difficulties' and values which emphasise being part of an inclusive society (Simons, 1992). Such a group reinforces the very category that people are seeking to downplay.

At the beginning of the 1990s, Simons (1992) noted few connections between self-advocacy and disabled people's groups. It is only recently that social model ideas about pride in a separate identity have begun to impact on the self-advocacy 'movement', with some more radicalised individuals challenging the dependence upon non-disabled allies which is characteristic of normalisation. This has been marked in debates over research ownership where Aspis (2000) has challenged the right of non-disabled individuals to undertake research into learning disability using the slogan drawn from the disability movement 'Nothing About Us Without Us'. At the time the social model of disability was being developed by disabled people, services for people with learning difficulties were largely influenced by normalisation, SRV and *An Ordinary Life*. As argued above, the chief strategy for change that arises out of these service ideologies is for people with learning difficulties to 'pass' into the non-disabled group. And the onus for making change is on professionals and communities. In contrast, the more politicised lobby of disabled people draws upon the social model of disability to raise the consciousness of all disabled people, with the intention of tackling disadvantage through political action (Oliver, 1990). The disabled people's movement tends to regard professionals with suspicion – the goal is empowerment of disabled people to take control of their own lives (Priestley, 1999).

The relationship that people with learning difficulties and self-advocacy organisations have had with the disability movement is not straightforward. Aspis (quoted in Campbell and Oliver, 1996) draws attention to the discrimination that people with learning difficulties have faced in the disability movement. People with certain impairments, including those with learning difficulties, are not always welcome. A degree of tension between people with learning difficulties and the disability movement is indicated in this statement from Swindon People First:

Disabled people without learning difficulties need to
- respect us,
- listen to us,
- learn from us and
- not lecture us and tell us what we should think (Swindon People First, 2002, p. 100).

Both Clement (2004) and Chapman (2005) in investigating the way self-advocacy groups operate found that where groups of (physically) disabled people became involved, there was often little respect for the distinctive perspectives of the members with learning difficulties.

At present it is hard to assess what impact the social model of disability has had on people with learning difficulties and their organisations. Pride in a different identity is not marked. Research that explores how people with learning difficulties perceive themselves suggests a very limited self identification as 'disabled'. Davies and Jenkins (1997) found that only 28 per cent of their sample of people with learning difficulties included themselves in the social category of people with mental handicap/learning difficulties and that 13 per cent of those discussed their identity in ways that were partial or unclear. Finlay and Lyons (2000) reported that it was hard to find evidence of a group identity, which they argue needs to be present if people with learning difficulties are to discuss and bring about change for themselves.

Some disability scholars have adapted the social model to consider the idea of 'internal oppression' that the attitudes of disabled people may themselves be self defeating (Shakespeare *et al.*, 1996). Drawing on the social model, one might argue that people with learning difficulties are subject to internal oppression, in which they absorb the devalued position that they as a group have in society and try to distance themselves from this negative identity. Todd and Shearn (1997) identified strategies used by parents to shield people from knowing that they were the possessors of a 'toxic identity'. However, this apparent failure of people with learning difficulties to claim some pride in their identity may be a factor of time. It may be worth considering the possibility that people with learning difficulties need the opportunity to learn about the social model before one concludes that it is an alien concept, imposed from afar.

Impact on policy and practice

The impact of social model thinking on learning disability policy and practice has been both direct and indirect. Legislation on Direct Payments and Disability Discrimination embraces people with learning difficulties although few have benefited (Morris, 2004). Independent living remains a dream for many people with learning difficulties. Environmental alterations such as ramps and wide doors, hearing loops and aural announcements on trains do also, of course, benefit some people with learning difficulties, but they do not address the barriers that a lack of literacy or social skills create for people's meaningful participation

(Walmsley, 1997). There have been efforts to create accessible forms of communication (*Valuing People* was available in a large print, simple language, illustrated format, as well as on tape), but these are largely confined to learning disability specific areas, rather than enabling access to mainstream culture, leisure and work. In a rather similar vein, academia has responded to the claims of people with learning difficulties to citizenship with a plethora of initiatives to engage people as collaborators in research projects and writing, with varying degrees of success (Walmsley and Johnson, 2003).

One of the most striking developments of the period was the emergence of groups, called 'self advocacy groups' which claimed to 'speak up' for people with learning difficulties. A further consideration of the ideas which have contributed to the remarkable rise of self-advocacy follows below. The social model has, however, had an impact on thinking in this area. Chapman's study of supporters working in five different self-advocacy groups across the UK suggests that both social model thinking and normalisation/SRV are present in the philosophy of such organisations. In the organisation most overtly committed to the social model there was a commitment to employing people on a full wage, in contrast to those where a more confused mix of normalisation, SRV and so-called People First thinking reigned. In those organisations there was a tacit acceptance that there would always be a need for non-disabled support (Chapman, 2005). Clement's (2004) study of another large English self-advocacy organisation suggested that close involvement with disabled people's organisations created a new form of hierarchical oppression by physically disabled people over members with learning difficulties.

Valuing People itself at first sight owes a debt to social model thinking. Unequivocal statements such as 'people with learning disabilities are citizens too' (DOH, 2001b, p. 9); 'all this can be done by believing that people with learning disabilities can move on and be more independent' (p. 9); and, perhaps most overtly 'you should be proud of who you are' (p. 10) can be read as statements compatible with the social model. However, in many respects, the prescriptions for improvement are not so influenced, with a great emphasis on improvement of person-centredness in services, prescriptions more readily associated with normalisation/SRV than the social model which has aspirations for full political and economic participation, well beyond the perspective of services.

In summary, the key differences between social model and normalisation ideologies are, first, that the social model places the responsibility to change with society rather than the impaired individual, whereas nor-malisation is ambivalent in this respect. Second that whereas normalisation's primary focus is on services, this is a secondary issue for the disability movement for whom the aspiration is beyond special services to personal assistance to allow individuals to pursue their own goals (Morris, 1993; Priestley, 1999). It is indeed difficult to envision a White Paper on disabled people equivalent to *Valuing People* emanating from the DOH or equivalent, for the use of mainstream health services, and the use of personal assistants takes disabled people, in theory if not in practice, beyond the purview of the care system. Such an analysis indicates why the social model has been less influential as an ideology in learning disability – it is hard to visualise a situation in which most people with learning difficulties could thrive without high quality services managed by a third party (Burton and Kagan, 2006). Indeed, any move to do so might indicate, not progress, rather a return to the neglect which was characteristic of services prior to the 1970s, and, as campaigns against the closure of traditional services have shown, would be vigorously contested by parents' groups (Concannon, 2004).

Self-advocacy

The idea that people with learning difficulties can be active contributors to debates about their interests rather than passive recipients of other people's care has been a key plank in the evolution of claims for citizenship status and may parallel the rise of parents' groups in the earlier period as the most significant new ideological development of the late twentieth century (Bersani, 1998). The earliest 'speaking up' events, in the 1970s, were organised by the CMH, an organisation of professionals and advocates committed to normalisation (Brandon and Ridley, 1985). A more detailed consideration of the evolution of self-advocacy will be found in Chapter 14. Here it is worth noting that the way self-advocacy developed in the UK was in contrast to its birth in Canada and Scandinavia where self-advocacy emerged under the wing of parents' organisations (Bylov, 2006; chapter 7). In the UK, independent groups, outside the service or traditional voluntary sector structures, rapidly became the gold standard, although latterly Goodley (2002) has argued that it is the style of support that is the salient factor, rather than its funding source.

Over its short life it is possible to discern a number of different, sometimes competing, constructions of self-advocacy. As Chapman (2005) has pointed out, there is an inherent tension between individuals using self-advocacy groups as a mechanism to gain confidence and skills in speaking up and self-advocacy organisations campaigning for change on behalf of the collective. Self-advocacy as a means of individuals gaining confidence requires a continual process of inducting and supporting new members, whereas if they are to be effective campaigning organisations, self-advocacy groups need people with experience and sophisticated skills in debate and management of budgets and people. These do not sit easily together.

In its early manifestations, learning the skills of 'speaking for yourself' dominated (Simons, 1992; People First, 1993; Atkinson, 1999). Slightly later came a trend identifiable in the literature as uncovering the authentic voices of people with learning difficulties. Atkinson (2002) links this to affirmation of identity and argues that there is a strong interrelationship between self-advocacy and life history research. This resulted in life story-based publications including autobiographies by Nigel Hunt, Joey Deacon, David Barron and Malcolm Burnside (1967, 1974, 1996 and 1991 respectively), and anthologies (Atkinson and Williams, 1990; Atkinson *et al.*, 2000; Traustadottir and Johnson, 2000). This self-advocacy-linked research contributed greatly to a broader understanding of how people with learning difficulties see and experience the world, not always as passive victims but also people with agency, feelings and relationships (Atkinson, 2002; Rolph, 2002; Johnson and Traustadottir, 2005). However, towards the end of our period, as the need to consult and involve users became a statutory requirement, individual 'speaking up' became increasingly marginalised. Rather these organisations became a vehicle for mobilisation of a voice that can speak for the collective (Buchanan and Walmsley, 2006).

Self-advocacy has also been acclaimed as a 'new social movement'. This position is most clearly articulated by Bersani. He claimed: 'whether we look for ideological change, revolutionary leadership, organising for power, the fact is that what we have come to call the "self advocacy movement" meets the definitions of a social movement' (Bersani, 1998, p. 61). Clement (2004) casts doubt on these claims. He contends that the campaigning element excludes the mass of people with learning difficulties whom the organisation claimed to represent and that there has been a great deal of 'talking up' self-advocacy with a sometimes rather optimistic focus on its potential as a transformative movement. There is, however, no disputing that its symbolic importance is enormous, if people with learning difficulties are indeed citizens, rather than recipients of care.

Conclusion

The role ideas and ideology have played in the shaping of community care has been the theme of this chapter. Although it is important to stress that ideas alone did not drive change, they did create mental frameworks within which change was conceptualised. There is, as the chapter has shown, a complex interrelationship between ideas developed and expounded by social researchers and theorists and their policy manifestations. Arguments put forward by normalisation and social model theorists have found their way into policy, in part for humanitarian reasons, though Andrew Scull's rather cynical interpretation that the ideas were used as a camouflage for cost-cutting has some validity.

Ideas associated with normalisation and SRV have been the dominant influences in thinking around learning disability, and, we would contend, continue to retain that position. Social model ideas have offered different tools for thinking, but, largely because of the nature of the impairments people with learning difficulties have, there has been far less progress towards models of assistance under the direct control of the service user (Emerson *et al.*, 2005). Accompanying the assertion of the rights of people with learning difficulties is an emphasis on individual rather than collective wellbeing, with much reliance on person-centred planning, Direct Payments, and access to work and employment, which some have begun to critique as overly dominated by individualised market-based models (O'Brien and Towell, 2003). In this latter respect, the shift from care to citizenship has dangers, in that its flipside could all too easily be neglect.

But this warning should not lead us to dismiss progress as an illusion. This review of the last 30 years of the twentieth century reminds us of the huge distance travelled conceptually. We have moved from Kushlick's cautious Wessex experiment to full inclusion for some children with special needs in schools, with appropriate assistance provided as of right, and a vision, for a tiny minority even a reality, of a satisfying life, fully supported by responsive personally controlled services. In this amazing journey, a debt has to be acknowledged to the influence of ideas.

Note

1. Oral history interview with the author, March 2005.

Part II
Organisations and Structures

Part II of the book describes the organisations and structures that were in place for people with learning difficulties in England between 1948 and 2001. It shows how policy slowly changed, from providing places in hospitals to providing community care through the establishment of hostels and Day Centres. It shows how the way things were done slowly followed changes in ideas and how many obstacles delayed change. In 2001, *Valuing People* set out a vision for services which promoted independence, rights and choice – a stark contrast with its 1971 counterpart which had better care as its guiding philosophy. Chapter 5 addresses organisations and structures in the three smaller countries of the UK: Wales, Scotland and Northern Ireland.

3
Organisations, Structures and Community Care, 1948–71: From Control to Care?

John Welshman

Introduction

This chapter moves from the theoretical to the practical, from the ideas and ideologies considered in Part I, to organisations and structures. It moves from what was said to what was done, taking up the challenge issued by Malin, Race and Jones to chart the reasons why each affected the other, but also to explore why they so rarely appeared to be in harmony (Malin *et al.*, 1980, p. 65). In terms of the implementation of policy, this section also offers an opportunity to test arguments regarding the development of services for other groups of service users. Robin Means and Randall Smith, for example, have argued that it is possible to see the period 1948–71 as one of incremental progress for domiciliary services for older people; the argument was over the respective roles of the state and voluntary organisations in service provision (Means and Smith, 1985, pp. 292–3). More recently, Anne Borsay has questioned how far community care policies were able to deliver social citizenship for people with disabilities by the late 1970s. She writes of the 1970 Chronically Sick and Disabled Persons Act that 'sustaining social rights was difficult where loss of autonomy was a precondition for the receipt of a service' and that social citizenship was attenuated with community care because geographical access to local authority provision remained highly variable (Borsay, 2005, pp. 169, 191, 196).

While the concept of community care remained ambiguous, in this period it referred to services provided by local authorities, and lacked the explicit reference to the role of the voluntary sector, the private sector and the family that was to become increasingly influential from the early 1980s. The Government conceived of community care as care outside the big institutions. Not until the 1970s was it reinterpreted as care by the community of relatives, friends and neighbours (Bayley, 1973, pp. 342–4; Digby, 1989, p. 93; Borsay, 2005, p. 180). Mental health and learning disability were often bundled together in both policy documents at the national level and service organisation at the local level, creating problems for the historian. Where possible, this chapter explores the implementation of care in the community through a more focused exploration of services for people with learning difficulties.

The period begins with the inception of the NHS in 1948 and ends with *Better Services* which signalled a clear policy intention to develop community-based services. In some respects, *Better Services* did reflect tentative moves towards a citizenship model, the third key theme of this book. Writing in 1975, Kathleen Jones saw the White Paper as heralding 'a move forward from the purely negative phase of preoccupation with abuse to a positive phase where new medical and social policy would create a better service' (Jones, 1975, p. 13). Nevertheless, it was a period when institutional provision was continuing to grow rapidly. The structure of the chapter is as follows. First, it describes interwar precedents for care in the community, before describing the situation in 1948, at a time when community services were extremely patchy. Second, the chapter traces the extent to which the changing ideas outlined in Chapter 1 were reflected in key policy documents – the 1954–57 Royal Commission; the subsequent 1959 Mental Health Act; the *Health and Welfare* White Paper (1963); and the 1971 White Paper. Third, the chapter explores the implementation of care in the community, focusing in particular on two aspects: the theme of work, as seen in Occupation Centres and JTCs and ATCs; and accommodation for adults, explored through the establishment of hostels. The chapter argues that although there were many delays in the implementation of a policy of care in the community in the period up to 1971, such changes as there were provide support for conceptualising the period in terms of a fundamental shift from an ideology of control to better care as the overall aim.

Earlier precedents for care in the community

As noted in Chapter 1, there are interwar precedents for care in the community, and many of the component parts of this policy can be grouped under the heading of an ideology of control. Earlier writers were eager to trace antecedents of the 1950s emphasis on care in the community in earlier provision. Writing in 1960, for example, Kathleen Jones argued that the 1913 Mental Deficiency Act, through provisions for guardianship, institutional care and licence, 'made it possible for many defectives to continue living in the community while still receiving a degree of care and control' (Jones, 1960, p. 72). Mathew Thomson has also suggested that shortcomings in the 1913 Act were overcome through using the voluntary sector to provide care in the community. There was a mixed economy of care in evidence before 1948, in which local authorities, voluntary organisations, hospitals and families themselves all had a role to play. Because services were only developed gradually, voluntary organisations in particular continued to have an important role. These included the Mental After-Care Association (1879); the Central Association for Mental Welfare (CAMW); the Child Guidance Council; the Order of St John and the British Red Cross; the Women's Voluntary Service; and the NSMHCA (1944). It was only in the 1950s that the local authority became the major provider and effectively had a monopoly on provision – though even in the 1950s voluntary groups set up nurseries, instituted holidays and leisure pursuits (Rolph, 2005a).

The number of mental defectives under the various types of care in the community, along with the fact that the Government itself was using the term by the 1930s, means it was possible to speak of a community care policy in the interwar period. Forms of community care included ascertainment, supervision, guardianship and licensing. In 1939, there were 40,000 'defectives' under statutory supervision; 26,000 under voluntary supervision; 4500 under guardianship orders; and 3000 on licence from institutions (Thomson, 1998a, p. 154). Thomson suggests that ideas of community were evident in institutional care – colonies and villas – while community care also adopted institutional models, particularly the Occupation Centres. Thus institutional and community care were closely linked, both ideologically and strategically. Overall the community care solution to the 'problem' of mental deficiency 'extended the influence of the institution into the community, and modified the nature of that influence' (Thomson, 1998a, pp. 149–79).

There were also experiments with hostels in the interwar period. The Wood Report (1929), for example, had argued that 'the hostel affords valuable training and an opportunity of testing the defectives' fitness for more responsibility and increased liberty' (Board of Education and Board of Control, 1929, p. 26). Moreover in 1923 and in 1930, Evelyn Fox of the CAMW turned to the idea, popular in America, of 'working hostels'. These were seen as providing an organised and supervised way back into the community from institutions and were regarded as a form of short-term provision (Rolph, 2000, pp. 9–10). Hostels were opened by some voluntary organisations. Eagle House, for example, was opened as a hostel for feeble-minded girls by the Surrey Voluntary Association for Mental and Physical Welfare in May 1924. Potential residents were to be 'of stable temperament, without serious physical disabilities, and suffi- ciently intelligent to be able to perform ordinary household duties without a very great amount of supervision'. Most 'girls' worked in domestic service, but the work for 'boys' was more varied – farm labourers, gardeners and carpenters. Given the emphasis attached to saving the money earned through work, it was argued that the hostel system 'while making for happiness and self-respect, should also prove an economical method of dealing with the highest-grade of mental defec- tives in the community' (Gibson, 1930, pp. 75–7).

However, while this work has placed the origins of care in the community in the interwar period, recent writers have also been cautious. Thomson has noted that while patients, families and local communities were involved in policymaking, certification reflected a desire to control sexually active females, delinquent males and unrespectable families (Thomson, 1996, pp. 207–30). Walmsley and Rolph have argued simi- larly that it is more helpful to regard institutional and community care as a continuum and suggest that some forms of community care were motivated as much by a desire to control as they were by a wish to provide care. Despite gaps in implementation, the 1913 and 1927 Mental Deficiency Acts created a framework of formal community care, with community care as adjunct rather than alternative to institutional care. This managed the space between the family and the institution, supervising those outside the institutions on licence and providing the evidence for commitment to an institution. While feminist research of the 1980s stressed the burden community care policies placed on the fam- ily, families had always been expected to manage long-term care. Overall, Walmsley and Rolph conclude that formal community care has long had elements of care and control, and it was a combination of protecting the community and protecting the individual that was the main motivation behind the 1913 Act (Walmsley and Rolph, 2001, pp. 59–80).

The Second World War was crucial for the development of services for older people (Means and Smith, 1985) and had a similar role for learn- ing disability. The Emergency Medical Service required the discharge of 100,000 patients from existing hospitals on the outbreak of War, and many of those discharged were people with learning disabilities (Humphries and Gordon, 1992; Gelb, 2004). The potential uses of hostels were further highlighted during the War, when the evacuation of schoolchildren drew attention to the psychological needs of children

(Leslie, 1939–41, pp. 307–12; Fox, 1940, pp. 97–102; Board of Education, 1947, pp. 64–70). The War in this respect did provide an experiment in the potential use of smaller types of residential accommodation. For adults, voluntary organisations such as the CAMW developed agricultural hostels for patients from the mental deficiency institutions who worked on the land to assist home food production (Lovejoy, 1972, p. 220; Thomson, 1998a, p. 273). The main response of the state to the issue of older people reflected concern about their impact on the morale of others (Means and Smith, 1985). Nevertheless as the War progressed, the humane treatment of dependent groups became an important symbol of post-Beveridge Britain. Voluntary organisations were able to argue for reforms in both residential and domiciliary services for older people (Means and Smith, 1985, pp. 25–67). In terms of learning disability too, welfare was an important symbol for postwar Britain, and further illustrates the shift from an ideology of control to an era in which ideas around care gradually became the dominant theme.

The situation in 1948 and the structure of the NHS, 1948–71

It is debatable whether the changes or the continuities were more apparent at the time of the establishment of the NHS, in July 1948. What the NHS Act meant in practice was that responsibility for what was termed 'mental deficiency' continued to be divided between the RHBs and the local authorities (Webster, 1988, pp. 327–9). In terms of hospital beds, the then current recommendations were that beds should be provided at the level of 2.0 per 1000 population in the case of mental deficiency. However at the end of 1948, nine RHBs fell below recommended levels, with the worst being the Newcastle and Sheffield regions. Most patients remained for life after admission (Welshman, 2005).[1] Section 20 of the 1946 NHS Act reiterated the responsibilities of local authorities under the Mental Deficiency Acts, 1913–38. They continued to operate the system of ascertainment, supervision, licence and guardianship set up by the 1913 Act.

But Section 28 of the NHS Act also stated that local authorities could 'make arrangements for the purpose of the prevention of illness, the care of persons suffering from illness or mental defectiveness, or the after-care of such persons'.[2] Section 28 represented an advance on the procedures of the 1930 Mental Treatment Act, since it created a legal basis for local authority provision of preventive measures and residential alternatives to hospitalisation. While it was permissive, it did include a

Ministerial power to mandate local authorities to take action by order. Nevertheless responsibility for services in the community remained confused, and this, along with the permissive nature of local authority services, led to local variations in the quantity and quality of services (Unsworth, 1987, p. 247). The significance of these local variations in implementation and provision are pursued further in Chapter 13.

In the late 1940s some local authorities appointed Mental Health sub-committees, to replace the Mental Deficiency Committees that had run services in the interwar period, and initiated comprehensive care.[3] Others were content to carry on with the statutory services, without attempting to do more than was required of them. Some began to co-ordinate services, and co-operate with the hospital sector, to ensure continuity of care, but others remained in comparative isolation (Jones, 1954). Local authorities were responsible for Occupation Centres, hostels, social clubs and after-care. Kathleen Jones noted of Lancashire in the mid-1950s that where hospitals were co-operative and local authorities energetic, there was a greater chance of resettling ex-patients, but while this was being done effectively in some areas, in others it was non-existent (Jones, 1954, pp. 34–55). The task was especially hard in local authorities that did not prioritise learning disability. Other work has confirmed that while some local authorities such as Somerset (Atkinson, 1997) had well-developed provision, others like Bedfordshire (Walmsley, 1997) had virtually nothing. The Ministry of Health conceded in 1953 that mental deficiency had been a new departure for many local authorities; there was no general body of professional and administrative experience; trained staff were 'scarce'; and progress had been 'slow and uneven'.[4]

The tripartite structure of the NHS remained unchanged until the 1974 health service reorganisation. The only major organisational change of this period was set in train by the Seebohm Report of 1968. The Committee recommended that areas of social and medical services should be co-terminous; services including ATCs should become the responsibility of the new Social Services Departments; and LEAs should become responsible for the education and training of all 'mentally subnormal' children and for JTCs (DHSS, 1968, pp. 116–17). The direct outcome of the Seebohm Report was the 1970 Local Authority Social Services Act, implemented in April 1971. This meant that the new Social Services Departments took over responsibility for the social services required by the 'mentally handicapped' from the local authority Heath Departments. Similarly, with the 1970 Education (Handicapped Children) Act, the JTCs for children excluded from the school system under section 57 of the 1944 Education Act passed over to the LEAs. Other than the new Social Services Departments, the period 1948–71 was characterised by organisational continuity rather than change.

The Royal Commission on the Law Relating to Mental Illness and Mental Deficiency; the 1959 Mental Health Act; and the 1962 Hospital Plan

The main policy document of the 1950s was the Report of the Royal Commission (1957). As we saw in Chapter 1, the Royal Commission embodied many key ideas about care in the community. It introduced new legal terminology; it made new administrative arrangements; it made recommendations on admission and discharge; and it established Mental Health Review Tribunals (Jones, 1960, pp. 178–203). Parents contributed to the work of the Royal Commission, whereas they were not consulted about the 1913 and 1927 Mental Deficiency Acts, and this involvement of 'consumers' was a distinct difference from interwar practice. The Royal Commission argued that services for 'mentally disordered' patients should be an integral part of the general health and welfare services. Hospitals would provide in-patient and out-patient treatment for those who needed specialist medical treatment or continual nursing attention. But local authorities would be responsible for preventive services and community care, including Training Centres, Occupation Centres, residential accommodation, hostels and general social help and advice. The Royal Commission noted that this would involve 'a considerable expansion of residential and non-residential community health and welfare services' (Royal Commission, 1957, pp. 17–18). All local authority services should be available to those who could benefit from them without the use of compulsory powers, and those with 'mental disorder' should have access to the general social services. There was increasing emphasis on treatment, training and social services that could be given outside hospitals or which made earlier discharge possible (Royal Commission, 1957, p. 207).

The Royal Commission had assumed that a 'fair share' of national resources would be allocated to the mental health services, as the development of services should be given a high priority (Royal Commission, 1957, p. 210). The Mental Health Act of 1959 repealed previous legislation and introduced a single code for all types of mental disorder. The annual reports of the Ministry of Health illustrate how the Act further raised the profile of care in the community in policy rhetoric. In 1959, for example, the Ministry of Health noted that the Act had laid the basis for the expansion of community care services – training and Occupation Centres; social centres and clubs; home visiting services; and residential homes and hostels.[5] In 1961, it argued further that the results of planning were beginning to materialise, with an increase in the number of buildings. Local authorities were widening the range of services for the mentally subnormal, with special facilities for the severely subnormal, such as special units in JTCs; there was more specialisation, with separate Centres for adults and children; and more attention was being paid to residential accommodation.[6] For Kathleen Jones, writing in 1960, the Act offered a 'new starting-point' where 'a major change in public attitudes had led in 1959 to a comprehensive Mental Health Act – a land-mark only comparable to the original Lunatics' Act of 1845' (Jones, 1960, p. 3).

The secondary literature on the history of care in the community, mainly focusing on mental health, has made much of the argument that one of the attractions was the potential for economies in the costs of institutional care (Sedgwick, 1982; Scull, 1984; Busfield, 1986). Certainly the Conservative Government of 1955–59 departed from the recommendations of the Royal Commission in failing to support the theoretical commitment to the shift to community services with specific capital grants to local authorities (Unsworth, 1987, p. 299). Thus in many localities there was little progress towards the goal of community care (Unsworth, 1987, p. 316). Charles Webster concludes that the attempt to accompany the 1959 Act with the launch of a sizable community care programme was 'an abject failure'. The health departments fell back on their customary piecemeal approach, making minor advances when the opportunity presented itself (Webster, 1996, p. 120). The policy of care in the community was attractive to the Conservative Right, which had promised economies in public spending (Unsworth, 1987, pp. 261–2). Enoch Powell's famous 'water towers' speech of March 1961 made it clear that the Government favoured a reduction in the number of hospital beds. At the annual meeting of the NAMH, Powell noted of the large institutions 'there they stand, isolated, majestic, imperious, brooded over by the gigantic watertower and chimney combined, rising unmistakable and daunting out of the countryside, the asylums which our forefathers built with such solidity' ('Everybody's Business', 1961, p. 351).

The Hospital Plan published in January 1962 envisaged that capital expenditure on hospitals would rise steadily to reach £50m a year by 1964, and a new network of District General Hospitals would be established. The Plan noted of mental subnormality that there were 1.3 beds per 1000 population and substantial waiting lists. However planners found it more difficult to estimate provision for the next ten years, owing to waiting lists, greater life expectancy and the expansion of community services and treatment (Ministry of Health, 1962, p. 5). The Plan claimed that services had grown rapidly, as reflected in the numbers receiving training in ATCs and JTCs; at the end of 1960, there were 468 Centres, with a further 350 planned, along with hostels and facilities for sheltered employment (Ministry of Health, 1962, p. 12). It observed of community care that 'everywhere the scope for further development is great' (Ministry of Health, 1962, p. 12) and also noted variations in the services provided by different RHBs. In the Oxford region, for example, planners had found that 'hospital development has not been able to keep pace with the expansion of population, and there are shortages particularly of maternity beds and of accommodation for the mentally subnormal' (Ministry of Health, 1962, p. 169).

The 1962 Hospital Plan created a network of District General Hospitals, marked the end of the era of 'make do and mend', and reflected the acceptance of a long-term programme of capital development for the NHS (Ham, 1981, p. 25; Mohan, 2002). However there is less evidence for expansionism than appears on the surface, and the Conservatives avoided action on hospital planning in the interests of holding down health expenditure (Webster, 1994, pp. 59–68). The Plan fell well short of the objectives of its originators, and in terms of individual projects and as a comprehensive planning exercise, it was 'little short of a disaster, the full ramifications of which are still largely unchronicled' (Webster, 2002, pp. 121–4). John Mohan concedes that the Plan rested on 'somewhat insecure foundations', and long-term planning had only partly filtered into the Ministry of Health and the NHS, creating technical weaknesses; it was 'both a milestone and a millstone' (Mohan, 2002, p. 129). Certainly the low level of expenditure on mental deficiency was noted by social scientists. In 1961, Richard Titmuss pointed out that expenditure by local authorities in England and Wales on all mental health and mental deficiency services increased from only £1.3m in 1949–50 to £3.5m in 1959–60, the latter figure equivalent to the compensation for fowl pest given to farmers. He furthermore suggested that 'to transform the bad old mental hospital into the therapeutic institution will be an expensive process' (Titmuss, 1961, p. 356).

Two White Papers: *Health and Welfare* (1963) and *Better Services for the Mentally Handicapped* (1971)

The main planning documents associated with the development of care in the community in the 1960s and early 1970s were the *Health and*

Welfare (1963) and *Better Services* (1971) White Papers. As the Hospital Plan had attempted for hospitals, *Health and Welfare* tried to plan the long-term development of the health and welfare services. It consisted of 48 pages, some photographs and 321 pages of local authority returns. In 1962, all local authorities had been invited to prepare plans for the development of services in the next decade. The Ministry admitted that since local authorities were independent 'no attempt was made either to indicate common standards to which the plans should conform or to suggest modifications before publication' (Ministry of Health, 1963, p. 2). The White Paper did provide useful evidence on the scale of provision. In 1961, for example, some 61,164 'mentally subnormal' in-patients were under the care of psychiatrists (4.3 per 1000 population); 7000 patients had been discharged; and 11,002 people were referred to local authorities which in total were providing services for 80,000 people (Ministry of Health, 1963, p. 23). The White Paper conceded that the large regional variations in referrals and in the number of people receiving services were due not only to local differences in the extent of need, but in needs that had not come to light (Ministry of Health, 1963, pp. 23–30).

What the ten-year plans were intended to mean is indicated in Table 1. What is clear from the plans is the emphasis on intended provision for children and the priority given to hostels. The total capital building programme was some £223.4m in the period 1962–63 to 1971–72. In general, the 1963 White Paper has not attracted the same degree of attention as the 1962 Hospital Plan. Writing in 1964, for example, Peter Mittler and J. H. F. Castell were critical of the ten-year plans, suggesting that they showed an insufficient awareness of the need to diversify training and care, and a lack of standards in hospital provision and the staffing of community services. Despite the success of the Brooklands experiment, there was little evidence that such units were

Table 1   Anticipated increase in provision for the mentally subnormal, 1962–72

	1962	1972	+ (%)
Training Centres for adults	281	483	58
Training Centres for children	345	424	81
Training Centre places for children	16,407	23,031	71
Training Centre places for adults	11,259	27,795	40
Hostels	47	464	1172

Source: Ministry of Health, 1963, pp. 366–7.

being established, either within hospitals, or in the local authority services (Mittler and Castell, 1964, pp. 873–4; Mittler, 1966, pp. 22–3). Kathleen Jones found from her research in 1972 that at first sight it seemed that many local authorities had fulfilled their ten-year plans. The total number of places available in one RHB, comprising 11 local authorities, was very close to the original projections, and six authorities had exceeded their targets. Overall, however, the plans of 1963 had been followed by ten years of patchy development. Most local authorities approached their original estimates, and some exceeded them, but the original estimates were in many cases pitched very low by the standards of the early 1970s (Jones, 1975, p. 162).

Health and Welfare encouraged a systematic approach to the development of services; it drew attention to norms which were presented as desirable targets; it gave local authority staff a basis on which to draw up plans; it strengthened claims of health and welfare services for a greater share of resources; and publication of the plans provided a means of comparing the intentions of local authorities (Ham, 1981, p. 166). Arguably what is most striking from the figures in *Health and Welfare* is the surprisingly high number of JTCs and ATCs in an era when the Government was allegedly not serious about care in the community. However while the White Paper amalgamated the plans of local authorities, it failed to provide a rationale for community care (Walker, 1982, p. 16; Allsop, 1984, p. 57). There was no attempt to ensure compatibility with the Hospital Plan, and achievement fell well short of the objectives (Lowe, 2005, p. 85). Charles Webster points out that the tabulations were a synopsis of local authority plans. It was a rudimentary planning exercise, since there were no costings, except quinquennial estimates for capital expenditure. He concludes that these limitations help to explain the obscurity into which the community care White Paper sank (Webster, 1996, p. 126).

The other main policy document of this period was the *Better Services* White Paper (1971). As was noted in Chapter 1, the growing critique of institutionalisation was augmented when the Ely Hospital scandal (1967) shone a spotlight on care in mental subnormality hospitals. The White Paper argued that the strengths and weaknesses of community services stemmed from their historical background, along with the priorities adopted by local authorities in the face of financial restraints. The new Training Centres and residential homes were of high quality, but only a small start had been made in providing training centres for adults, residential care for adults and children, and practical help and advice for families with 'mentally handicapped' members living at home (DHSS, 1971, p. 13). The White Paper suggested that despite the progress made by local authorities, there were still serious shortages of facilities and staff, and the developments recommended by the Royal Commission 14 years earlier were far from being accomplished (DHSS, 1971, p. 18). Overall, it argued that no new policy was needed for local authority services; what was needed was faster progress to overcome the deficiencies, which would require more money and trained staff. It made an assessment of the number of places required for both children and adults per 100,000 population, thereby making it possible to make a more rigorous assessment of the level of provision. Thus 1800 places for children had been provided in 1969, against 4900 required. For adults aged 16 and over, 4300 places had been provided in 1969, against 29,400 required (DHSS, 1971, p. 42).

The White Paper has been interpreted as being partly a defensive move owing to the Ely Hospital scandal, and expenditure commitments were relaxed, although with specific targets and norms. Little of the policy was new; rather the White Paper reflected the determination of Keith Joseph (1918–94), Secretary of State for Health and Social Services, to make more rapid progress towards the objectives outlined by the 1954–57 Royal Commission (Webster, 1996, pp. 402–5; Webster, 2002, pp. 78–80). Kathleen Jones argued at the time that because the publication of the 1971 White Paper came shortly after the creation of Social Services Departments, it made comparatively little impact and was only 'an expression of general intent' (Jones, 1975, p. 155). What is most interesting to explore is what the implications of this slow development of services were for individual families in different parts of the country. This is what we seek to achieve in Part IV.

Assessment: Occupation Centres, JTCs and ATCs

The chapter now explores the development of services in the period 1948–71 through two themes: that of the establishment of Occupation Centres and Training Centres, and the broader theme of work, and the provision of local authority hostels. Although occupational health is of increasing interest for historians of medicine, the functions of work for people with learning difficulties have, with some exceptions, been ignored (Rolph, 2000; Walmsley and Rolph, 2001, pp. 72–4). Nevertheless work is of importance to our overall themes of care, control and citizenship. Anne Borsay, for example, has written that 'social citizenship was an empty promise for the many disabled people who were not properly integrated into the labour market' (Borsay, 2005, p. 139). The type of work that was provided, and the meaning of work itself, has important implications for the arguments that there occurred a fundamental shift from control to care, or that changing ideas about the nature of work were an important element in the emergence of citizenship.

In the late 1940s and early 1950s, the development of JTCs and ATCs proceeded very slowly, with curbs on capital spending holding up development of these alternatives to larger institutions. In some local authorities, Occupation Centres were a prominent feature of provision. In the interwar period, where they existed, they enabled children who might otherwise have been placed in institutions to live at home with their families and were part of the arrangements that kept people under surveillance (Walmsley *et al.*, 1999, p. 191). In the late 1940s, Occupation Centres for children were typically located in church halls. The children were usually engaged in handicrafts – sewing for girls and rug-making for boys – what were deemed 'useful occupations'. In November 1949, for example, the organiser of an Occupation Centre in Leicester wrote that 'happiness and discipline are my chief aims in the running of the Centre, as without these nothing can be achieved'.[7] Provision tended to lag behind need – the numbers attending the Occupation Centres were much greater than they could cope with. Despite shortages of building materials and restrictions on capital expenditure, some local authorities had managed to replace these with purpose-built Special Schools by the mid-1950s. Even so, the emphasis of the curriculum continued to be on 'industrious activity' such as repairing chairs, making benches, marking ambulance blankets and cookery classes (Rolph, 2005a–e).

At the national level, policy documents stressed the potential role that Training Centres might play. The Hospital Plan noted variations in local authority health and welfare services by region, including the number of people receiving training in JTCs and ATCs (Ministry of Health, 1962, pp. 278–9). Similarly, the *Health and Welfare* White Paper stressed the importance of Training Centres for children and adults, envisaging an increase in the number of places from 27,666 to 50,826, and from 626 to 907 Centres (Junior and Adult combined) (Ministry of Health, 1963, pp. 366–7). Ironically, the best-known workshop was not run by a local authority, but by the NSMHCA in Slough (Baranyay, 1971). In 1966, Peter Mittler wrote that 'one can only hope that the Slough experiment will set the example to be followed by those hospitals and local authorities who are as yet unaware of the possibilities of industrial training of the severely subnormal' (Mittler, 1966, p. 20). As we saw in Chapter 1, there was much emphasis in research studies by the Clarkes and others on employability and the potential for people to be productive citizens.

Even though they were initially housed in unsuitable buildings, Occupation Centres for children were a recognised element in local authority provision. In contrast, the equivalent services for adults were noticeable by their absence in most local authorities in the 1950s. By the early 1960s in some local authorities there was interest in what was being done in other countries. Staff from Leicester, for example, made visits to other European countries that were perceived as providing more 'progressive services'. In Holland, they found that workshops provided activities that included addressing envelopes, welding, sewing pyjamas, making boxes, assembling chairs and soldering. Holidays and recreation facilities were also provided at social centres.[8] Nevertheless back in Britain, in most local authorities, Occupational Centres for adults, now called ATCs, developed much more slowly compared with those for children, and, where they did open, the focus up to the early 1980s was on an industrial model that included laundry work, horticulture and other industrial pursuits (Carter, 1981). The delay meant that many adults aged sixteen and over remained in the Special Schools or in Occupation Centres for children, which had long waiting lists and were generally overcrowded.

While ATCs were transferred to Social Services Departments in 1971, the reality of life inside them was exposed by the Kathleen Jones survey. Most development that had taken place had been since 1967, and Jones reported a striking contrast between the newer purpose-built Centres and the older ones. The adult trainees in some respects got the worst of both worlds; denied the facilities thought appropriate for children, they did not have the freedom given to independent workers. Most of those attending Training Centres seemed to have little hope of finding outside employment; two-thirds did not have skills that would make them immediately employable (Jones, 1975, p. 164). Jones found that most of the work done was industrial, and of an elementary and mechanical kind. Around three-quarters of the total trainee population was engaged in tasks such as assembling and packaging simple pieces of equipment, such as telephone connectors. Contract work was difficult to obtain, and much work was dull and repetitive, providing little opportunity for moving trainees on from simple tasks to more complex ones. The male and female sides of Centres usually operated on highly differentiated lines, and there was little opportunity for parents to discuss the progress of their own children (Jones, 1975, p. 166). Machinery for woodwork, metalwork and laundry was often obsolete, and staff claimed that the pressure of contracts meant that there was not enough time to teach patients how to use equipment. Jones concluded that 'the result was a system which sometimes bears more relation to the nineteenth-century concept of "setting the poor to work" than to modern ideas of social development' (Jones, 1975, p. 167).

Oral history interviews have also helped to uncover the meaning of work more generally. Sheena Rolph, for example, has found from research on two hostels in Norfolk, Eaton Grange (1930) and Blofield Hall (1951) that work served many different purposes. While work at Eaton Grange provided a means to cross boundaries, access to wider social networks and a means to gain independence, it also served as an instrument of punishment and atonement, exploitation and a means of control (Rolph, 2000, p. 184). For men at Blofield Hall, work was more varied than at Eaton Grange, was enjoyed by many, and could act as a progression route. However at the same time, the emphasis on earning one's way out of the hostel hinted at the theme of atonement (Rolph, 2000, pp. 304–6). Getting people to make an economic contribution to society, or at least to defray the costs of their own care, has surfaced consistently – and was still part of policy rhetoric around proposed reform to Incapacity Benefit in 2006 (Welshman, 2006b). Overall, there was much evidence that attitudes towards work showed important continuities with the interwar period; the main aims of the Training Centres were economic rather than social. The emphasis again illustrates the pervasiveness of an ideology of control in which work was synonymous with supervision and surveillance. It was only in the 1970s that work came to be seen as a social good to be aspired to, as reflected in the enthusiasm for 'supported employment'.

Assessment: inside the walls of the hostel

While residential care has attracted much interest, with some notable exceptions the place of the hostel in community care policy has generally been ignored, in favour of a more general treatment of national policy and its implementation (Atkinson, 1998c; Rolph, 2000; Borsay, 2005, pp. 171–2; Welshman, 2006a). We have already seen how hostels were pioneered in the interwar years. In the postwar period, the growth of hostels coincided with the revival of a familial discourse, and a familial model became popular for many different groups (Rolph, 2000, pp. 44–5). The *Piercy Report* (1956), for instance, found a need for additional hostel accommodation for the disabled, including as both short-stay hostels for people leaving hospital and permanent hostels for the 'dependant disabled' (Ministry of Labour and National Service, 1956, pp. 29–30). The need for hostels was also stressed in the evidence received by the 1954–57 Royal Commission (Royal Commission, 1957, pp. 211–18). The *Health and Welfare* White Paper noted that the main thing was that the hostel should be like a real home. Foster homes or lodgings might be the best arrangement, but premises built or specially adapted as residential accommodation for the mentally disordered could be suitable, if the location had been chosen carefully and the premises were suitably designed and run (Ministry of Health, 1963, p. 25).

In some respects, the 1971 White Paper reflected new thinking, particularly in relation to creating 'family' type environments. Thus it argued that the term 'home' should be used in place of the word 'hostel', noting that the word 'hostel' had a ring of impermanence and a certain austerity, denoting a place where people stayed while working or studying away from home. In contrast, residential homes were a permanent substitute family home for most of the residents, even though they kept in touch with their own families and visited them as many times as possible. The White Paper argued that the staff and residents should become a substitute family group, and 'the home should be homely' (DHSS, 1971, p. 35). Homes should supply most of the residential care needed, and they should be small, with residents of both sexes. Maximum sizes were set at 25 places for adults, and 20 for children, and most adults should have single rooms, with no room having more than four beds. There should be plenty of space for recreation, both indoors and outdoors. The White Paper noted that 'in such surroundings a family atmosphere can be created, where individuals can develop within a small group and with their own interests and possessions' (DHSS, 1971, p. 35). However, much of this was aspirational and it conceded that most local authority hostels did not have this homely atmosphere. The emphasis on hostels in *Better Services* can be seen as progressive when compared to the large institutions, but as more limited when compared to group homes or supported living arrangements advocated later in the century.

The extent to which the aspirations of the White Paper were met can be gauged through contemporary social surveys. Kathleen Jones's 1975 survey found that hostels ranged from institutions with dormitories, hospital beds and low standards of furnishing to small establishments with a more homely atmosphere. Overall, there were three main types of accommodation – converted mansions; purpose-built hostels; and council houses. The converted mansions were generally the least suitable, being large and gloomy, and set in extensive grounds. The purpose-built hostels, despite having better facilities, were often rather clinical in character. The council houses were small and homely, but lacked facilities. No one pattern of accommodation was ideal for all types of residents.

Compared to hospitals, hostels had a relatively unregulated social life; with efforts being made to keep rules to the minimum necessary in a small community. Though one hostel 'looked like an outdated hospital, the corridors being badly lit and in need of a coat of paint, while the chilly lounge had shabby armchairs arranged in rows', others provided warm and cheerful environments (Jones, 1975, pp. 176–7).

Oral history interviews have also helped to uncover the reality of life in hostels. Sheena Rolph, for example, has found from her Norfolk hostels that they were seen in many different ways. At Eaton Grange, the presence of choice in everyday affairs and a degree of self-determination was confirmed by the reports of the Visitor, and this predated the normalisation theories of the 1970s (Rolph, 2000, p. 161). After the 1959 Mental Health Act, the idea of the hostel as a permanent home became less important than its role as a half-way house between the hospital and the community, and as a stepping stone to freedom. Similarly for men at Blofield Hall, the hostel acted as both a home for men going out to work and as a stepping-stone for those on their way out on licence. Efforts were made to transform the hostel into a more 'normal' environment, with the provision of sofas, a television and a bar, but tensions between care and control remained unresolved. Overall, Rolph has argued that 'hostels were a distinctive part of provision with their own ideology and role, not just small replicas of hospitals' (Rolph, 2000, pp. 315–19; Chapter 13). Nevertheless the work of Kathleen Jones and others provided important evidence on the reality of life in hostels and other forms of residential care, which again provides an important check on assumptions that there was a marked improvement in accommodation. Drawing on the language of the Wood Report (1929) which had argued that residential institutions should be 'not a stagnant pool, but a flowing lake', Jones concluded that there still were stagnant pools (Jones, 1975, p. 185). The language of the 1920s appeared to be equally applicable to the early 1970s.

Conclusion

This chapter has explored the implementation of care in the community, focusing in particular on two aspects: work, as seen in Occupation Centres, JTCs and ATCs; and accommodation for adults, explored through the establishment of hostels. The chapter has demonstrated that care in the community was only implemented patchily in the period up to the mid-1970s. It was a period when institutional provision was continuing to grow rapidly. Moreover the reality of provision in the mid-1970s was exposed by the research of Kathleen Jones and others, indicating important continuities in attitudes to work; in the provision of hostels and other types of residential accommodation; and in social work services and patterns of referral. Services had been slow to improve due to economic and attitudinal factors; money was required and people with learning disabilities remained a low priority in the eyes of the public. Thus despite the intention of the 1971 White Paper to create a situation in which hospitals were no longer custodial institutions, and the resources of health and social services could be brought to bear on the needs of this group of people, there was much evidence that the problems remained as intractable as ever.

Overall, however, the chapter has argued that although there were many delays in the implementation of a policy of care in the community in the period up to 1971, such changes as there were provided support for conceptualising the period in terms of a fundamental shift from an ideology of control, evident in the period before 1948, to an era when the development of facilities, albeit slow, had better care as its guiding light. This chapter has argued that in the period 1948–71, care in the community was increasingly prominent in legislative terms and as policy rhetoric. This is evident in such well-known policy documents as the 1954–57 Royal Commission; the subsequent 1959 Mental Health Act; and the 1963 and 1971 White Papers. All these bore the imprint of the ideas and research that were discussed in Chapter 1. The next chapter will explore policy and implementation through a study of structures and organisations in the period 1971 to 2000. In Part IV, the implications of the slow development of services for the experiences of individual children and adults, and their families are considered, as is the question of change and continuity in the workforce.

Notes

1. Sheffield Regional Hospital Board, *Quinquennial Report, 1947–52* (Sheffield, 1953), pp. 40–1.
2. 9 & 10 Geo. VI, *Public General Acts and Measures of 1946, National Health Service Act, 1946*, Chapter 81 (London, 1947), pp. 1119–214.
3. Leicester Health Committee, *Annual Report of the MOH, 1950* (Leicester, 1951), pp. 32–6.
4. Ministry of Health, *Annual Report, 1953* (London, 1954), p. 139.
5. Ministry of Health, *Annual Report, 1959* (London, 1960), pp. iv–v.
6. Ministry of Health, *Annual Report, 1961* (London, 1962), pp. 75–6.
7. Leicestershire Record Office, Wigston, Leicestershire (hereafter LRO): Leicester Mental Health Services sub-committee minutes, 1 November 1949.
8. LRO: Leicester Health Committee minutes, 18 November 1960.

4
Organisations, Structures and Community Care, 1971–2001: From Care to Citizenship?

Jan Walmsley

Introduction

This chapter examines organisations and structures during a momentous period in learning disability history. Organisations and structures alone can be rather dry, so the chapter's theme will be the extent to which citizenship was furthered by the various frameworks in place. We are discussing a basically positive period in learning disability history. As we will see from the life stories in Part IV, it was a period when life improved overall for people with learning difficulties, when people had greater opportunities for an ordinary life, and social inclusion, and when citizenship emerged as a policy theme. It saw the virtual ending of large state-run long-stay hospitals as a residential option and the inclusion of children of all abilities in mainstream schools as an attainable goal. However, the chapter will also explore some considerable continuity beneath the rhetoric of policy. The authors of the 1971 White Paper said of their proposed shift from hospital to community care that 'no new policy is involved for local authority services. What is needed is faster progress to overcome the present deficiencies' (DHSS, 1971, p. 43). Similarly, in 2004, a review of independent living and community care concluded that whilst much of the policy framework was in place to offer independent living to disabled people, including people with learning difficulties, there were major organisational, financial and atti-tudinal barriers to achieving the vision for individuals (Morris, 2004). Moreover, although it was a period of intense optimism, of a belief that the disadvantages of impairment could be overcome if the right policies, services and attitudes were in place (Walmsley and Johnson, 2003), the same problems as have dogged learning disability policy and services remained, with commentators dubbing some of the aspirations articulated in *Valuing People* 'romantic'. That is, that they represent a model of individualised consumer choice which was ill-suited to the needs of many people whose impairments would always render them vulnerable without strong societal support.

Conservative administrations dominated in the UK for most of the time. The Tories came into power in 1970, governed for four years before losing to Labour, and were then re-elected for 18 years of Tory rule, 1979–97. In 1997, 'New Labour' swept into power, and it was under this Government that *Valuing People* was initiated and implemented. It was also under this administration that devolved administrations in Scotland and Wales took over the administration of social care, leading to slightly different policies. However although both the 1971 and 2001 White Papers were born under Labour Governments, the political colour of administrations appears to have had relatively little impact. Like other social care groups, people with learning disabilities have been affected by the 'neoliberal turn' (Jessop, 1994), where Government drives to develop markets, encourage welfare to work and create individualised models of 'choice' in services, and several commentators have observed marked continuities between Conservative and New Labour policies in relation to social care (Grover and Stewart, 1999).

The chapter opens with a discussion of the realignment of learning disability policies, from an association with mental health to a much closer association with disability, and its consequences. The timeline on pp. xiii–xxi illustrates the legislative landmarks, alongside Government changes. It then gives an overview of the major policy directions of the period, particularly the shift from 'health' to local authority controlled services which accompanied the big change, deinstitutionalisation, followed by a brief description (with examples) of the marked rhetorical shift, from a philosophy of control and care to one where the emphasis is on rights. The introduction from 1990 onwards of care management is examined. The following section examines in microcosm developments in two important areas – day services and education. Next, the rise of two consumer groups is considered – carers and users – as a feature of developments which have impacted upon the organisations and structures supporting community care. This is contrasted with the rediscovery of abuse as a significant factor impacting on people's lives, one which points to the importance of retaining 'care' alongside citizenship if people with learning difficulties are to enjoy a reasonable quality of life. Finally, the chapter ends with a more detailed comparison of the 1971 and 2001 White Papers, and the contexts in which they were written.

Learning disability, mental health and disability

As is illustrated in Chapter 1, there has been a lengthy association between mental health and learning disability in terms of policy and practice. Not only did the 1959 Act legislate for both groups, Duly Authorised Officers (DAOs) and Mental Welfare Officers (MWOs) were charged with the supervision of both groups in the community. Rolph, Atkinson and Walmsley have shown that mental health usually got priority, and oral evidence reiterates this. Stephen Thornton commented that 'when you combine mental health and learning disability, mental health always takes the time, the crises, staff shortages, patients who threaten violence. Learning disability just trundles along'.[1]

In the period after 1971, policies for learning disability and mental health diverged significantly, in contrast to the earlier period covered in Chapters 1 and 3. Whilst the White Papers of 1971 and 1975 (*Better Services for the Mentally Ill*) had many similarities, not only in name, but in their commitment to running down long-stay hospital care in favour of community-based services, by the end of the period there was divergence, with learning disability policy becoming more benevolent and rights-based while that for mental health laid, if anything, greater emphasis on control than its predecessor of 1913. The timeline shows the significant policy initiatives, but there will be little in this chapter on mental illness, specifically, because it had become less of an influence on learning disability policy and practice. The shift of services for learning disability decisively into social care as opposed to 'health' in the late 1990s, while mental health remains a primarily health service-staffed function, has further enforced the growing divide.

As the chapter on ideas and ideology in the period 1971–2001 has shown, there were mixed blessings in the association with (physical) disability ideas given the stress on individuals controlling their own care, but overall this pushed policy in the direction of citizenship rather than control, with legislation to permit access to Direct Payments being the most obvious example. In many respects, mental health policy went in the other direction with, at the time of writing, mooted changes pushing more for control and the undermining of human rights (Sainsbury Centre for Mental Health, 2005). The realignment is well illustrated by changing terminology. The language used has changed frequently. The language of 'mental subnormality' was replaced, first by 'mentally handicapped', the term used in the 1971 White Paper, then by 'people with a mental handicap' and then (around 1990) by 'people with learning disabilities' (the Government's preferred term) or 'people with learning difficulties' (the term preferred by user groups). The linguistic shift from labels which include 'mental' to labels which include 'disability' is virtually complete, and while language does not necessarily drive change, it does reflect changing ideas (Walmsley, 2001).

The big change: deinstitutionalisation

If it is remembered for anything in learning disability, the last 30 years of the twentieth century will be remembered as the period when most of the large hospitals closed. Although institutional care had been widely criticised since the NCCL campaign of the early 1950s, as Chapter 1 shows, in practice the long-stay hospitals had continued to expand in numbers, albeit gradually, until the late 1960s (DHSS, 1971, p. 19) giving the NHS a near monopoly in residential provision. Indeed, several major hospitals actually opened in this period. It took a long time for the institutional momentum to slow down. Although the 1971 White Paper did not visualise the closure of long-stay hospitals, in the period 1971–2001 those community care solutions advocated throughout the preceding half century became a reality on the ground.

Perhaps equally momentously, responsibility for learning disability services shifted from the central government via the NHS to local authorities as a result of the 1968 Seebohm Report (DHSS, 1968). This was an extremely slow process, with 'health' hanging onto a significant role through its running of hospitals and involvement in provision of residential units, and through the influence of learning disability nurses and some psychiatrists who continued to claim professional hegemony over learning disability. Money played a part. As the House of Commons Social Services Committee Report on Community Care put it in 1985, 'the fundamental reason for the NHS becoming increasingly involved in community based provision for mentally handicapped people is that they have the funds and local authorities do not' (Sinclair, 1988). By the end of the period, however, responsibility for learning disability was firmly in social care, whether provided by the private, voluntary or state sectors (Means *et al.*, 2003), although commissioning (formerly called purchasing) of services was a joint responsibility between health and social care, and, confusingly, health could also be a provider if a health body successfully tendered to run a service. Ironically, although this has effectively challenged the medical hegemony, it may have in other ways been detrimental as health services, particularly from 1997, benefited from vastly increased funding whilst social care has been starved of resource (Means *et al.*, 2003).[2] The location of learning disability in social care is not entirely secure – recent proposals are but the most recent of a series of identified threats to social services as the 'lead agency' for community care (Means *et al.*, 2003).

The large NHS hospitals were replaced by a host of community-based hostels, later group homes, supported living, independent living funded through Direct Payments, supported employment, along drives to improve access to leisure, to friendships and to sexual relationships. In sum, these were associated with the type of life most people took for granted, an 'ordinary life' (King's Fund, 1980). Fashions about the type of accommodation thought appropriate also changed, with smaller units increasingly preferred over large. Whereas in the 1970s large hostels were the norm, by 1988 the Wagner Review of Residential Care was of the view that 'although new hostels are still being planned and built, it could be that the present generation of purpose-built hostels is the last. There is a growing feeling that a buildings based service is inflexible' (Atkinson, 1988, p. 127). These predictions proved accurate. Hostels fell into disfavour, and the later 1980s, 1990s and early twenty-first century saw trends to smaller units – group homes for up to seven people, individual flats and even owner-occupied houses for some under shared ownership schemes. These developments in residential care are well illustrated through the individual life stories highlighted in Part IV, Experiences.

The main beneficiaries of the thrust to residential care were the residents of former hospitals. The Wagner Report (1988) noted that little progress had been made towards providing for people who had remained with their families, thus:

> There is now an accumulation of adults, some middle aged, with ageing and elderly parents, whose futures are still unplanned and uncertain, and who are at risk of being admitted to a residential setting during a major family and personal crisis. (Sinclair, 1988, p. 131)

Not much changed in this regard. It was estimated in 2005 that 29,000 people lived at home with parents over 70 (*Viewpoint*, 2005, p. 18). Similarly there was in 1988 little opportunity for young people to leave home as they reached adulthood (Sinclair, 1988, p. 131). A lack of statistical data makes it hard to establish a clear picture, though anecdotal evidence suggests that parents in 2005 expected that provision for residential care would be made as their young people approached adulthood (Dumbleton, 2005).

Not only were people living with families not catered for, there has been an increasing acknowledgement that the specific needs of families from black and minority ethnic and cultural groups have been neglected. Following a number of key studies which researched the experiences of such groups (Shah, 1992), concerns began to be voiced regarding the double discrimination often encountered. Families' experiences of being socially excluded by language barriers and racism, negative stereotypes and attitudes (Baxter *et al.*, 1990; Mir *et al.*, 2001) have emerged as important issues for policy makers, most noticeably in *Valuing People*. However, although there is at the policy level a greater awareness of the needs of people with learning difficulties from Black and Minority Ethnic (or other minority) groups, there is little in place to ensure that steps are taken to address the issues (*Viewpoint*, 2005).

Economic factors

We have seen in earlier chapters that the changes in the form of care were partly explained by changes in ideology, but economics had an important role in pushing governments and local authorities towards deinstitutionalisation. Not only did poor levels of funding help create the conditions which discredited hospital care, as highlighted by the Ely and other reports, but also community care was expected to be less expensive (Dalley, 1989). As Stephen Thornton put it in his interview, 'it was a Western world belief that this was the right thing to do and policy makers jumped on the back of it because it was cheap'.[3] Together, these push and pull factors help explain the momentum behind deinstitutionalisation.

In the 1970s, spending on mental handicap lagged well behind spending on health services for the general population. In 1975–76, for example, per capita funding on beds in mental handicap hospitals was £8.96 per day, compared to between £20.37 and £31.41 in acute hospitals (Ryan and Thomas, 1987, p. 167). Institutions were increasingly catering for more severely handicapped patients which also increased costs; at the same time the number of mildly handicapped patients who had earlier assisted in the running of the hospitals had dropped (DHSS, 1971, p. 19).

The 1971 White Paper set aside cash for improvements in community services, £40m for each year 1971–75, but ominously intoned 'the main responsibility lies with local authorities themselves', given that, as it said 'no new policy is involved for local authority services' (DHSS, 1971, pp. 43–4, paras 198, 206). No money was ring-fenced for the expansion

of learning disability services which meant that, as ever, they were subject to considerable local variation.

During the 1970s, hospital closures moved very slowly. Whereas in
1971 there were 58,850 people in hospitals, this figure had fallen only to
51,500 in 1980 (Wright *et al.*, 1994). Stephen Thornton is insistent that
closure was not envisaged, though improvement was. He recalled, 'we
were interested in the quality of care in the institution, we needed to
sort that before setting up lots of mini institutions in the community'.[4]
One of the major barriers to closure was financial. Not only was it
almost as expensive to run a half-full hospital as it was to run a fully
occupied one, it did not benefit local authorities who were therefore
unable to adequately fund new services. Cash savings from hospital
closures accrued to Health Authorities whilst the cost fell on local
authorities (Johnson, 2005). It was the 1980s which saw acceleration so
that by 1990 there were 32,700 hospital beds, 37 per cent fewer than in
1980 (Wright *et al.*, 1994). The acceleration is explained in part by financial factors. The 1981 Community Care Act addressed the perverse
incentive which rewarded health for closure and penalised social services.
At the same time, changes in the rulings governing board and lodging
allowances in 1983 allowed the use of social security payments to fund
places in voluntary or private-run accommodation if the person could
show financial need (Johnson, 2005). As a consequence, public expenditure on private residential care increased from £10m in 1979, to
£1872m in 1991 (Means and Smith, 1994). This led to rapid development
in the so-called mixed economy of care – the number of beds in voluntary
organisation-run homes for people with learning difficulties increased
by 271 per cent between 1980 and 1990 (DHSS, 1980; DOH, 1990,
quoted in Wright *et al.*, 1994). In effect, residential care was being paid
for by the social security budget, not health or social services.

The Audit Commission was critical of this new 'perverse incentive',
reporting in 1986 that it encouraged excessive use of residential and
nursing home care. Whilst this was often detrimental to the welfare of
older people, the perverse incentive does appear to have created the
impetus for large numbers of people to leave large long-stay institutions,
to be resettled in hostels and later group homes (Audit Commission,
1986). Money continued to be an issue throughout the period and
undoubtedly will be so for the foreseeable future. Government-funded
research has shown that high quality community care is not cheaper
than hospital care. Researchers found that while some types of living
accommodation were cheaper than a hospital place, on average new
types of accommodation were more expensive. At 1992 prices, hospital

had cost an average of £514 per person per week, whilst after five years, average costs for the same population in community-based housing was £598 per person per week (Cambridge *et al.*, 1993, p. 72). Local authority responsibility for learning disability services has meant that there has continued to be a wide variation in the type and quality of services available, and the pace of change has been inconsistent (Fryson and Ward, 2004).

Furthermore, financial pressures on the private care sector have led to many smaller providers going out of business, to be replaced by larger firms. In 1992 there were only six private sector providers with 1000 beds or more; in 1998 there were 17 (Laing and Buisson, 1998, 1999). This has implications for service user choice.[5] Further individualisation of care services, under schemes like Direct Payments, are argued by governments to be cost neutral, though it is argued that 'deconstructing a 20 bed care home offering 24/7 intensive support and dispersing that into 20 individual services will require more money, staff time and adapted housing stock' (Churchill, 2005, p. 18).

Markets, quasi-markets and care management

One major development in terms of organisation was the shift from monolithic provision of services by the NHS or Social Services to the creation of purchasers (later commissioners) and providers of services initiated by the 1990 NHS and Community Care Act. This was one of the most far-reaching and significant organisational changes of the period, affecting all health and Social Services activity. In 1971, virtually all services were directly provided by statutory agencies, funded either by taxation collected by central government in the case of health, or local taxes (successively rates, Poll Tax and Council Tax) in the case of Social Services. This change has been described (Means and Smith, 1994), but warrants some space here because of its profound impact on the lives of people with learning difficulties.

The 1990 Act is one of the landmark pieces of legislation behind the organisation of community care. Although it draws on the moral superiority of community care ideas (Walmsley, 1997) it was in large part motivated by the need to curb social security payments for residential care. The open-ended, nationally funded and controlled Department of Social Security budget for care was replaced by a cash-limited, locally administered budget only for those users who were individually assessed as requiring support. Purchasers purchase care on behalf of clients who have been assessed as requiring them. The services are provided by organisations which tender under a competitive process (initially

Compulsory Competitive Tendering, subsequently Best Value) for the privilege. Thus a quasi-market is created. The rhetoric of choice has been extensively deployed to justify this marketisation, though outwith Direct Payments the link between consumer preference and the service provided is often hard to discern (Walmsley, 1997).

None of the three women whose life stories are featured in Part IV mentions choosing her service or service provider. This is done on behalf of individuals by care managers, drawn from a number of existing professional roles (such as social work and nursing) who undertake the assessment, hold the budget and negotiate the care package. Where block contracts are negotiated for a large number of places in care homes or in day services, the semblance of choice is even less convincing, given that in any specific area there are likely to be large-scale providers who dominate provision. Since the introduction of the quasi-market in the 1990s, there have been further developments which emphasize consumer sovereignty. Although hearing service users discussing the price of housing is a marked advance in terms of social inclusion and citizenship, there are indications that people living alone in their own homes can be left to cope with minimal support services, and if they do not have reliable support from family or friends can struggle with maintenance.

Direct payments are, at the time of writing, a favoured policy direction. In their pure form, Direct Payments remove cash from the control of the service-based care manager into the hands of the service user who then decides how to spend the money and who to employ. Choice is elevated to a position above all others. Direct Payments have made little progress for people with learning difficulties (Swindon People First, 2002; Morris, 2004), and, for all but the most able, they present clear challenges in implementation without considerable support from family, friends, advocates or service providers. They have also been criticized as creating personal assistant jobs which are non-unionised, lack opportunities for career development and training and have little protection from the vagaries of individuals with little experience of acting as employers (Bornat, 2005). Nevertheless, at the time of writing, a new Adult Social Care Green Paper visualises individual control over budgets and care services as the way forward. In such a scenario, care services become services deployed in support of individual citizenship.

Policy impacting on children: from exclusion to inclusion

If for adults the period is characterised by deinstitutionalisation, the promotion of 'an ordinary life', and an increasing emphasis on citizenship and rights, for children it saw a long overdue ending of hospital care, and an increasingly vigorous debate over the advantages and disadvantages of integration or inclusion in ordinary schools. The 1971 White Paper, for example, records shamefully that there were 6400 children in hospitals in 1969 (DHSS, 1971). The absolute right to a full education for all children without exception was only established in England and Wales by the 1970 Education (Handicapped Children) Act. This finally brought all children, no matter what their disability or degree of learning difficulty, within the framework of education. For the first time, children with learning difficulties were embraced by the school system. No longer were those deemed ineducable excluded from school, confined to local authority-run JTCs or inadequate hospital schools. A 100 years after universal elementary education was introduced, everyone was entitled to a school place. Michael Tombs (parent) viewed this as the single most important change during his son's lifetime (born 1961) because it meant children were visible as they travelled to and from school (Rolph *et al.*, 2005, p. 278).

A medical framework in the form of the 11 categories of handicap of the 1944 Education Act continued to dominate special education, however, until the Warnock Report (DES, 1978) sought to replace this with a more educational framework. Many of Warnock's recommendations and ideas made their way into the 1981 Education Act, including the concept of a continuum of need rather than categories of handicap, and an educational definition of special needs and learning difficulties. The Warnock Report also raised the profile of early intervention, recommending that the education of under-fives with special educational needs should be a priority area. The concept of investment in the early years as a preventive measure proved to be a lasting one, reiterated in the Green Paper *Excellence for All Children* (DfEE, 1997).

Following the 1981 Education Act, children and young people defined by the law as having 'special educational needs' were given a number of entitlements. Most significantly, they were entitled to have their needs identified, to be formally assessed for a statement of special educational needs, to have provision set out in any statement of 'special educational needs' and to have the statement regularly reviewed. This legal entitlement was extended to under-fives. The Act also introduced a legal duty on LEAs to place children identified as having special educational needs in mainstream schools, though this duty was qualified by three conditions or 'caveats', any one of which LEAs could cite as a reason for placing a child in a Special School. The 1993 and 1996 Education Acts endorsed these caveats. It was not until the 2001 Special Educational Needs and

Disability Act that two of the caveats were removed, thus creating a strengthened, though still qualified, right to a mainstream placement, which can only be denied on the grounds of incompatibility with the efficient education of other children. The disability provisions of the Act make it unlawful for schools and LEAs to discriminate against disabled pupils, in particular in relation to admission arrangements and the educational provision offered at school. With the disability anti-discrimination legislation now extended to schools, colleges, universities and providers of adult education, the 2001 Act gave parents new rights of appeal to the renamed Special Educational Needs and Disability Tribunal, if they felt that a disabled child had suffered discrimination.

The history of education in this final part of the twentieth century is one of increasing access to education, ultimately within mainstream schools. As with adult services, the discourse has changed from needs to rights, influenced by the international drive for inclusive education as articulated in the Salamanca Agreement. Any assumed notions of straightforward progress, however, may disguise the realities of families' and pupils' varied experiences with schools as providers of education, support, stigma and inclusion or exclusion, issues which will be touched upon in Part IV. The debate over special versus mainstream schooling continues to overshadow education for children with special needs, with some parents vociferously objecting to the closure of Special Schools, while Government policy remains firmly in favour of integration/inclusion in mainstream schooling. In fact, Baroness Warnock has gone back on her earlier commitment to mainstream schooling, saying that it was not always appropriate.[6]

Day services: organisational change in microcosm

Day Services for Adults is an organisational area which well illustrates the ways in which services developed during the period. The aspirations are for full inclusion, citizenship rather than care, but the reality is somewhat less clear. Deinstitutionalisation pushed the creation of Day Centres, but their existence preceded it. If people were in hospital, then community-based Day Services were not required. But hospitalisation had never been universal. Mencap estimates that at its peak only half of the adults with learning disabilities were in institutions (quoted in Walmsley, 2000a). Other than staying at home with families, or the very slim chance of paid work, daytime occupation was a necessity if community care was not to rely entirely on the family. The 1971 White Paper recommended that there be 1.5 Day Centre places per 1000 population (DHSS, 1971). Of all its recommendations, this was the one that appears to have been most rapidly adopted. Day Centres (otherwise known as Occupation Centres, later ATCs) had existed since the inter-war period, but their growth was more pronounced following the White Paper. A survey published in 1981 states that three out of every five 'Centres for the Mentally Handicapped' had opened since 1970, with the average size of Centres increasing from 85 in the 1960s, to 120 in the 1970s (Carter, 1981). The 'golden age' of Day Services growth was 1960–76, with about 46,000 places for mentally handicapped adults being created. Unlike other client groups, Centres for the mentally handicapped at the beginning of the 1980s were almost exclusively the preserve of Social Services Departments (Carter, 1981, p. 57), thus being paradigmatically illustrative of the significance of local authority provision in learning disability community care. Also, unlike other client groups, there was an aspiration of a Day Centre place for all eligible adults (Carter, 1981, p. 168) and that it should be a 5-day a week full-time placement.

At the time of Carter's survey, the big emphasis in Day Centres was on contract work such as packing crackers, assembling electrical components, laundry work, horticulture and gardening. In some cases for those most able this was combined with domestic training – learning to clean, cook, make beds and generally conduct a normal life. Carter expressed several concerns about the way Centres were organised and run, including the dangers of a new form of community segregation; the permanency of some placements; the segregation of staff and clients; lack of choice, activity, even of what food to eat; and poorly-trained staff, many with a background in industrial rather than care work. In some Centres, she observed the continuation of institutional practices of physically segregating men and women in corridors, workshops and eating places. She concluded by asking whether the Centres' *raison d'etre* was not more control than care or development (Carter, 1981).

In the decades following this survey, changes in Day Centre philosophy were quite profound. Even in 1981, Carter found a Centre in Stockport which was experimenting with an individually tailored skills-based programme, allowing 'users' to move out from a home base to experience different environments and learn new skills such as photography, baking, language and self care. A positive expectation that users would move on was an aspect she singled out for praise in contrast to the more traditional 'place for life' approach of mainstream Centres (Carter, 1981). The type of provision being pioneered in Stockport became the norm in Centres now labelled SECs during the 1980s, with less emphasis on contract work and more on 'education for life'. In the early 1990s, researchers found that most ex-residents of mental handicap hospitals used segregated facilities – ATCs, SECs – where they received training in life skills and crafts as well as leisure activities and social clubs. They reported that 90 per cent of users enjoyed going to Day Centres and enjoyed the company of those they met there (Cambridge *et al.*, 1993, p. 67). The DOH encouraged the trend 'to shift away from services based on the traditional Adult Training Centre'. Buildings need not be abandoned, advised a circular, but could be converted to a resource centre. The main thrust of policy should, however, be geared to the use of integrated facilities – schools, colleges, recreation facilities, social clubs, cinemas and open spaces.[7]

Writing in 1994, other observers commented that 'the implementation of these policy guidelines is bound to occur gradually because of the resource implications ... day services are moving to a more intensively staffed form of provision than existed in SECs' (Wright *et al.*, 1994, pp. 35–6). These words are prescient as, although there has been a signifi-cant increase in attendance at Colleges of Further Education, the trend to 'services without walls' remains aspirational rather than real in many areas, with considerable scepticism amongst family members that it is anything other than a cost cutting exercise. Nor is it hard to find service users who have spent four decades in Day Centres and who can relate their history through personal experience as well as any historian!

'Users' and 'carers'

A significant element of the organisations and structures of community care in this period was the incorporation of 'carers' and 'users' into its fabric. Chapter 14 will touch on these issues in relation to the role of the voluntary sector in community care. As far as carers are concerned, there was from the 1980s an increasing awareness of the 'burdens' of having a child with a learning disability. Public and professional attention had hitherto tended to focus on the movement of people from hospital to community, obscuring the reality that over half the adults with learning disabilities in Britain live, and, throughout the last century, have always lived with their families (Sinclair, 1988; Walmsley *et al.*, 1999). Policy interests in community care and its implications for families prompted research. Attention was particularly directed at mothers, and their plight was highlighted in a number of research studies (Bayley, 1973; Glendinning, 1983; Ayer and Alaszewski, 1984; Abbott and Sapsford, 1987).

It is apparent that carers became of greater interest to policy makers because of the move to community care and that the research described above gave insight into what policy makers might do to support them. Whereas in the period before the Second World War families were closely regulated for their ability to control the behaviour of their offspring with learning difficulties, the postwar period saw their rehabilitation as heroes deserving of both pity and, later, support (Walmsley, 2000b; Walmsley and Rolph, 2001; Rolph *et al.*, 2005). The community care reforms of 1990 made informal family carers a centrepiece of policy. The DOH noted that 'the reality is that most care is provided by family, friends and neighbours' (DOH, 1989, para. 2.3). Thus supporting informal carers became a recognised element of social provision, with the DOH stating that:

> The Government recognises that many need help to manage what can be a heavy burden. Their lives can be made easier if the right support is there at the right time, and a key responsibility of service providers should be to do all they can to support and assist carers (DOH, 1989, para. 2.3).

This, of course, did not emerge from a vacuum. Feminists had campaigned alongside pressure groups such as the National Association of Carers for recognition of the unpaid work of family carers (Bytheway and Johnson, 1998). However, the 1990 reforms, for the first time, explicitly recognised the importance of this informal support. The outcome was legislation directed to support family or informal carers – the 1995 Carers Recognition and Services Act – and the development of services such as respite care and domiciliary care specifically aimed at making caring responsibilities more bearable. Thus family carers became part of the organisations and structures which support community care. The degree to which this was effective is debatable. Research into the experiences of families with severely disabled sons and daughters suggested that services remained disjointed and inadequate (Hubert, 1991; Burke and Signo, 1996). Meanwhile press reports of the struggles of families, some quite dramatically tragic, continue to surface, as do gaps in services.[8]

The impetus for the incorporation of the user movement into the fabric of community care was rather different. The user movement of people with learning difficulties began in the UK around the mid-1980s with the establishment of People First London Boroughs. A survey undertaken in 1989 found a considerable number of groups, some 'independent', that is, supported by advisors who were outside services, but many were part of the service system in ATCs and residential care (Crawley, 1989). The user movement in learning disability has been associated with the broader Disability Rights Movement which began in the 1970s, with the struggle for self-determination and an end to 'dependency born of powerlessness, poverty, degradation, and institutionalisation' (Charlton, 1998, p. 3). Disabled people led a campaign for disability rights legislation arguing, via the social model, that it is society, and not a person's impairment, that is disabling (Finkelstein, 1980; Oliver, 1983). The vocabulary of services, and of people's expectations, became more rights based. The right to Direct Payments won in legislation in 1996 can be attributed to effective campaigns by disabled people and their organisations, something from which a few people with learning disabilities benefited.

Self-advocacy organisations have to a limited extent followed the lead of disabled people's organisations in demanding and expecting rights for people with learning disabilities, and for them to be at the centre of the decision-making process, as illustrated by slogans such as 'We are the Experts' and 'Nothing About us Without Us' (Chapman, 2005). However, in-depth research into these organisations suggests that the degree to which their agenda is controlled by their members as opposed to paid supporters is often limited (Clement, 2004; Chapman, 2005). Furthermore, demands on them made by services often make it difficult for them to single-mindedly represent what their members want, as opposed to meeting the need for services to demonstrate consumer representation (Concannon, 2004).

The role of users has been enhanced by Government interest in supporting a consumer voice in the development of policy and the running of services. This accompanied the marketisation of services in the 1990s, with service users redefined as consumers or customers (Davies *et al.*, 2005). In line with a general move to increase the 'user' or 'patient' voice in the development of services, the Government has been broadly supportive of this development. The active inclusion of people with learning difficulties in the development and implementation of *Valuing People* is the most obvious manifestation of the recognition of the user movement, and Government's positive stance towards it.

There has been criticism of the incorporation of the self-advocacy movement into the organisations and structures of community care. The requirement of *Valuing People* for representation on Partnership Boards (DOH, 2001a) has intensified the workload for organisations representing people with learning difficulties, without any obvious practical benefit to the majority (Fryson and Ward, 2004). Issues of representation remain fraught with difficulty, particularly as only the most able and vocal of service users are able to participate meaningfully, and their ability to effectively speak for others, often more severely disabled, has yet to be proven (Concannon, 2004). Furthermore, 'carers' and 'users' do not often speak with one voice. Indeed, there appears to be an inherent tension between the interests of family members in protecting their sons and daughters (care), often through the maintenance of paternalist service models (such as full-time placement at Day Centres), and the demands of the more radical end of the user movement for independent living (citizenship). Several studies indicate that parents are weary of consultation and fear that change actually means less resource (Tilley, forthcoming; Concannon, 2004), a debate also echoed in education over the closure of Special Schools.[9] User organisations rarely express such concerns as clearly, though there are indications that the value people accord to their current services is greater than the rhetoric implies (Rolph and Walmsley, 2006), with the role they play in sustaining friendship networks being particularly important (Walmsley, 1995a; Rolph *et al.*, 2005).

The (re) discovery of abuse

Perhaps ironically, as the carers' and self-advocacy movements gained strength, so did a parallel, but oddly disconnected, campaign to command the recognition of the abuse of people in service settings. Led by researchers such as Ann Craft and Hilary Brown from the early 1990s, this movement reinvigorated the 'care' rhetoric, that is, it was not enough to convey rights if people did not have the capacity to be heard or protected. Serious shortcomings in services were highlighted by investigations such as the LongCare enquiry, and some put the incidence of abuse of women with learning disabilities as high as 80–90 per cent (McCarthy, 1998). The Government responded with the policy guidance *No Secrets*, and some efforts to strengthen court proceedings so that people with learning disabilities could give evidence with more chance of being taken seriously. There has, however, been little impact to date as courts fail to recognise evidence given by people with learning difficulties as valid. A protracted struggle over new capacity to consent legislation is a manifestation of a clash between the 'rights' based arguments of People First and the 'care' based arguments of parents groups, and others. Perpetrators of abuse have been explicitly identified as staff and other residents (Brown and Barratt, 2002). They have rarely been the families which remained the darlings of social policy, despite evidence from a number of research studies featuring the 'voices' of service users that their families had been far from havens of love and security (Rolph and Walmsley, 2006).

From *Better Services* to *Valuing People*: A comparative analysis of the White Papers

This period, 1971 to 2001, is framed for England by the publication of the two White Papers. This chapter ends by comparing them. As we have noted, it was a period when 'community care' finally triumphed as a policy option, both in rhetoric and in reality, and during which public perceptions of learning disability were at their most optimistic for well over a century. The aspirations of people with learning disabilities to be taken seriously, to be active citizens participating in society and to have a voice both reached the surface and were to some extent fulfilled during this period. Whereas in 1971, the fight was to close hospitals and replace them with hostels and Training Centres (for adults) with a strong 'care' message, and the views of people with learning disabilities were assumed, by 2001, those views were actively canvassed in the preparation of, and follow-up to, *Valuing People*. It is, in short, a quite remarkable story of change.

The background to the White Papers differs. Whereas *Better Services* was in part prompted by revelations of appalling neglect and abuse in long-stay hospitals, which had brought services for people with learning disabilities into the media eye, and put pressure on the Government, by the end of the twentieth century, learning disability was more of a policy backwater. There are indications, however, that this was a success for a group of academics and professionals who had been looking for mechanisms to hasten reform, and who finally found a responsive minister. Civil servants had been making the case for a new strategy in a relatively low key manner to John Hutton's predecessor as Minister of State at the DOH (Paul Boateng) who was reported to be fairly receptive to the idea. Hutton therefore arguably inherited the idea and perhaps saw it as something that was fairly easy to start up and show early delivery in his tenure in the Ministerial role.[10] The other important point to note is that it was originally only a strategy, and not a White Paper. As such, it was fairly low profile, low risk. It was only when it became clear that the work had substantial support from the learning disability field, and would be seen as a positive news story, that there began to be political support for its being a White Paper.[11]

In the light of our citizenship theme, it is worth pointing out that the development and writing of the *Valuing People* strategy was the first attempt by Government to include the voices of carers and individuals with learning difficulties. A Task Group was set up of people with learning difficulties who travelled the country visiting self-advocacy groups and collecting evidence of the quality and often, disparity, of local services. Following on from the launch of the strategy, a National Forum of people with learning difficulties was set up with four representatives elected to the Task Force, the body set up to oversee the implementation of the strategy. This put the voice of people with learning difficulties into the centre of the government process. The force behind *Valuing People* was therefore the active engagement with carers and people receiving services in the development of national policy and the encouragement at the same time of an inter-departmental approach to moving services for people with learning disabilities onto a more mainstream basis. The strategy represented a change in attitude to 'person-centredness', and a more participative approach to policymaking.

Just as their antecedents and mode of development were very different, the White Papers look very different. *Better Services* is an A5 paperback pamphlet, under the *imprimatur* of the DHSS and the Welsh Office. There is no attempt to make the text inviting or accessible. There are no illustrations, other than tables. *Valuing People*, on the other hand, is A4 size with full colour photos of smiling people of different ethnic backgrounds and varying degrees of impairment on its cover. Although the main version contains no further illustrations, the print is two colour, with liberal use of summary boxes. Furthermore, there is an accessible version, also available on tape, illustrated with colour cartoons of the type commonly in use at the time, intended to help people with learning difficulties access the printed word. In terms of content, rather than style, there are also stark differences. The most obvious are that, whereas in 1971 the emphasis was on expansion of services, particularly those outside long-stay hospitals, in 2001 it was on the *improvement* of services, to make them more person-centred.

As far as the themes of this book are concerned, *Valuing People* came out championing 'Rights, Independence, Choice, and Inclusion' (DOH, 2001a, p. 3). The 'citizenship' word is not used specifically in this slogan, but there are clear connections between Marshall's concepts of citizenship and the 'rights' of the White Paper. While both White Papers commit to greater spending, their objectives bear close scrutiny. The first and second objectives of *Better Services* (to explain why services needed to be extended and improved and to invite greater sympathy and tolerance on the part of the general public for the 'mentally handicapped') were closely linked to a 'care' theme. The aims of *Valuing People* are not set out as clearly. Rather we are presented with 'A New Vision' and some aspirations which might loosely be called aims. Under the overall heading of 'Better Life Chances for People with Learning Disabilities', we find

- more choice and control for people with learning disabilities,
- supporting carers,
- improving health,
- housing, fulfilling lives and employment and
- quality services (DOH, 2001a, pp. 4–8).

This quite marked difference in approach carries through into the body of the White Papers. *Better Services* is a lengthy document which attempts to set out the situation regarding services in some considerable detail. Whilst one might take issue with the medical framing of some of the data, and the prescription of types of service – no acknowledgment of ethnic diversity, no aspirations for supported living or employment – it is undeniable that setting out an evidence base of whom we are talking about, and what their needs may be, is reassuring. In effect, *Better Services* set out some concrete objectives for local authorities, namely 43,500 more places in ATCs than were in use in 1971; 24,100 residential places for adults; and 2800 for children (DHSS, 1971). We know that these targets were not met in the timescale set (see above). They did, however, set up a major expansion in provision of Day Centre and community-based residential placements.

Valuing People had a more challenging job if it was attempting to map provision, for, whilst in 1971 there were few providers which were not either NHS or local authority, by 2001 services were provided by a bewildering array of organisations – private, voluntary and statutory, not to mention hybrids such as Direct Payments, or family carers. Its authors made little attempt to chart this complex picture. Whilst it is stronger on values than its predecessor, *Valuing People* is surprisingly devoid of statistics (DOH, 2001a, p. 15, figure 1). Far more data were available by then in other formats, for example, the comprehensive DOH website. However whereas in 1971 there were clear and measurable targets for what was then regarded as improvement, in 2001 any target was vaguely worded, and by any standards hard to measure. Probably the most concrete performance indicator in the White Paper is the aspiration to empty NHS long-stay hospitals by April 2004. This was achieved, though not by the target date. Moreover although commendable, this has not necessarily led to community inclusion or participation for all those who might once have found themselves in hospitals. It also does not address those long-established institutions run by non-NHS bodies which continue to flourish to this day. This means that for some, citizenship is an abstract and distant goal – care and control remain the philosophy.

Conclusion

This chapter has been an overview of the organisations and structures, primarily in England and Wales, which supported community care for people with learning difficulties between 1971 and 2001. It has, of course, told an over-simplified story. As other social policy analysts have pointed out, the pace of change has been such that it is hard to write a coherent account of policy changes (Means *et al.*, 2003). The extent to which the evolution of policy impinged on the lives of the families will be considered in later chapters where accounts from different stake-holders, including families and 'users', help us to resist the assumption of a notion of progress, where *Valuing People* represents the triumph of liberal values. Rather we are more hesitant about the idea of 'progress', acknowledging that while some 'improvements' have been made, in other respects the picture is more mixed. For many, particularly those with more severe impairments or with 'challenging behaviour', there was less change. This is a theme that has been touched on in this chapter and will be revisited in Part IV, particularly the service users' accounts.

Notes

1. Interview with the author, March 2005.
2. *Community Care News*, 7–13 July 2005, p. 6.
3. Interview with the author, March 2005.
4. Ibid.
5. Personal communication with the editors.
6. *Guardian*, 31 January 2006, Education section, p. 5.
7. DOH circular, 1991.
8. *Guardian*, June 2000; *Observer*, 23 February 2003.
9. *Guardian*, July 2005.
10. Personal communication with the editors.
11. Ibid.

5
Devolved Policy for People with Learning Difficulties in Scotland, Wales and Northern Ireland

Rohhss Chapman

Introduction

When discussing health and social care policy in the United Kingdom, there is often a focus on England, largely due to the historic power of Westminster. This chapter seeks to overview the policies of the different Parliaments of the UK, thus redressing the balance. Indeed it is argued that there is a lot for Westminster to learn from policymaking influenced by local and regional issues. Defining what exactly makes up the UK is contested. Payne and Shardlow (2002, p. 21) point out that the 'historical entanglement of the countries of the British Isles has left a complex set of interwoven constitutional arrangements'. For the purposes of this chapter, the UK is described as the countries of England, Wales, Scotland and Northern Ireland. The picture is actually more complicated than this when considering the partnerships and effects of other crown dominions such as the Isle of Man and the Channel Islands. The Isle of Man Parliament, the Tynwald, predates the Parliament at Westminster and was a construction of earlier ties with Norway, whilst Eire has embraced the EU to the extent of adopting the euro. Our history within the British Isles is therefore highly complex.

After the 1946 NHS Act for England and Wales, followed by the 1947 NHS Act (Scotland) and 1948 Health Services Act (Northern Ireland), there were three main Departments set up to be responsible for health and social care in the UK at the local level (see Part II). These were Health, Welfare and Children's Departments. These Departments were essentially responsible for care services for people with learning difficulties. By 1971, they had been consolidated into Social Services Departments in England and Wales, and into Social Work Departments in Scotland. This paved the way for the change from specialist to generic social services, although there were always specialists operating within generic teams. When these Departments were formed, the idea was to work together with health services. By 1979, the Jay Report argued that people with 'mental handicap' should live in the community and receive support from social rather than medical care professionals. The pledge to community care was consolidated in *Care in the Community* (DOH, 1981). This chapter sets out to describe the administrative structure in each country and then focuses on a discussion of the differences and commonalities of themes around social policy and care for people with learning difficulties in each of the countries of the UK, drawing out the main aspects of difference and commonality.

Devolved government, current context and policies that affect people with learning difficulties

Devolved government in Scotland, Wales and Northern Ireland has developed and changed over the period analysed in this book. However, defining devolution is also problematic. Ideologically there are two main perspectives: first, that devolution is about descent to regional government through a series of changes (the core to the periphery) (Hechter, 1975); or second, that devolution is about the lapse of an unexercised right to the ultimate owner (e.g., the Scottish Nationalist view). Interestingly the *Oxford English Dictionary* defines devolution as 'the moving of power or responsibility from a main organisation to a lower level' – or from a central government to a regional government. These arguments about the meaning of devolved power link into issues around identity, inclusion and nationalism. Issues around national identity appear as an often understated but important factor in the relationships between each country of the UK. As Payne and Shardlow comment, 'a key element in the construction of this state was subjugation by the English of the other nations within the British Isles' (Payne and Shardlow, 2002, p. 20).

Parliament based at Westminster in London, has, as noted, directed most government activity for the UK. However the arrangements of administration and services for people with learning difficulties in Scotland, Wales and Northern Ireland are distinctive in a variety of ways. Each country has a Secretary of State and an administrative department located in the Central Government (London). Each country also has its own assembly (elected members) and administration, which take on the work of specific departments (based in Edinburgh, Cardiff and Belfast). Laws which apply in Scotland and laws that apply in

Northern Ireland differ from the law in England and Wales, which are historically more closely linked.

Policy that affects the lives of people with learning difficulties therefore differs slightly in each of the countries, although they have a number of common underlying values such as person-centred planning, rights, independence, choice and inclusion (Scottish Executive, 2000; DOH, 2001a; JRF, 2002). The Disability Rights Movement which began in the 1970s heralded the rise of the self-advocacy movement in the UK (Rolph *et al.*, 2005). Subsequently, all current policies acknowledge the importance of advocacy in its different forms. In all countries at the moment, apart from Northern Ireland, a common feature is that for the first time Government has funded advocacy and therefore acknowledges the influence and impact of the 'service user' movement. The policies that currently directly relate to the lives of people with learning difficulties in each of the countries are:

Scotland	*The Same As You?* (May 2000)
Wales	*Fulfilling the Promises* (2003)
Northern Ireland	*A Review of Mental Health and Learning Disability Services (Northern Ireland)* (2002).

Scotland

Out of the three countries, the Scottish Parliament has the most extensively independent role, running its own civil service and deciding on its own social policy. From the 1970s, the campaign for a Scottish parliament stressed the inclusive, civic sense of being Scottish (Kiely *et al.*, 2005, p. 150), where Scottish national identity has always been a key issue (Hearn, 2000), interfacing with much of the policy and decision making taken by the Executive. The powers granted through the devolution process, when the Scottish Parliament was formed in 1999, largely governed social welfare where there was already a degree of Scottish autonomy (Stewart, 2003).

Most decision making (apart from legislation about regulation and abortion) has been devolved to the Scottish Parliament in Edinburgh. The Scottish Executive Health Department is responsible for the leadership of the NHS and putting into practice the policies relating to health and community care. There are 15 NHS Boards responsible for the delivery of Care and Community Health Partnerships in each area of Scotland. In the broader context, Scotland provides free social care and yet (or perhaps, because) poverty is currently viewed as a major problem in Scotland. The health of the population of Scotland is worse than either that of the populations of the rest of Great Britain or Europe on a range of indicators, with a fifth of the Scottish population living in income poverty (JRF, 2005).

In Scotland, *The Same as You?* (May 2000) was issued before *Valuing People* (2001). The review was the first in-depth analysis of services for people with learning difficulties in Scotland for over 20 years. It took an inclusive approach, by involving statutory agencies, 'service users', their carers and people who deliver services. It gathered information about social and health care services for adults and children with a learning difficulty, with a view to developing more innovative and person-centred services. After the review, a 'blueprint' for services was set out for the next ten years. Scotland People First were involved as part of the Parliament's inclusive approach. Similar to *Valuing People*, there was much concentration in the policy document on person-centeredness and the importance of self-advocacy. Scotland People First, based in Edinburgh, were funded to develop groups around the country to represent their views. This illustrates the link between policy and the focus on services. Indeed Scotland People First comments that all of its work focus can be traced back to elements in *The Same As You?* (Chapman, 2005).

However there are some notable differences between the Scottish and the English experience around the closure of long-stay hospitals. According to Waterhouse and McGhee (2002, p. 151), the Day Centre attendance of people with learning difficulties had changed little since 1990, which suggested that the long-stay hospitals had also taken longer to close than in England. The hospital closure date in England was March 2006, but in Scotland it was predicted that by the same date, there would be 17 people left in long-stay hospitals with 109 people 'undetermined' (Scottish Executive, 2004). Partly the problems in Scotland have been located in the difficulty of finding appropriate places for people to move in to. Because of this, one of the recommendations of the Scottish Executive was to ensure adequate advocacy involvement. The Chairperson of People First Scotland had a vision that a UK People First self-advocacy movement should be formed but acknowledged that there were difficulties in getting each country involved. Ironically, Scotland and Wales had been successful in creating national advocacy organisations whereas England had been unable to achieve agreement upon how it could most effectively work (Chapman, 2005).

Wales

The Welsh Assembly, also set up in 1997, has its own Parliamentary body but less of a role (than Scotland) in determining its own legislation. The National Assembly for Wales has strategic responsibility for the NHS in Wales. The Local Health Boards are statutory bodies responsible for commissioning and putting into practice local healthcare initiatives. Specialist services for people requiring more complex care are provided by Health Commission Wales. Each Local Health Board responds to one of three regional offices. These offices are charged with assessing and reviewing the development of local health and social care plans.

Ely Hospital in Cardiff was the focus of allegations of abuse of people with learning difficulties in the *News of the World* in 1967 (see Chapter 1), but despite this, specific policy for people with learning difficulties had an auspicious history in Wales. As mentioned in Chapter 4, the AWS (1983) marked a departure from the concept that having a learning difficulty was an illness, thus moving away from the medical model. There were five key concepts, which ran through the AWS, which are still uppermost in policy today. These are: participation, representation, equality, choice and satisfaction. The AWS was viewed as a continuation of ideas, which had been difficult to implement, from the *Better Services* White Paper.

Hunter and Wistow (1987, p. 10) commented how conventional wisdom dictated that the Welsh Office would have an essentially reactive role, taking its lead from the DHSS in London rather than developing an independent initiative of its own. However this was clearly not the case with the AWS. In explaining the specific circumstances which led to the formulation of the AWS, an important aspect had been the small administrative machinery required for a population of only 2.8m, which set Wales apart again from the other separate offices of Scotland and Northern Ireland. Because personnel could be based in one building, Hunter and Wistow reflected that a culture of informal teamwork was nurtured along with continuity of staff through promotion. The important special demographic features of Wales, the rural communities which upheld traditional culture and especially the Welsh language, were compounded by specific working conditions. This led to an energetic and high profile approach to new services (Hunter and Wistow, 1987, p. 10). Also significant was an attempt to redirect a perceived imbalance of service for people with learning difficulties following the slow progress towards deinstitutionalisation set out in the 1971 White Paper. This was one of the outcomes of the Special Conference in Cardiff to discuss services for 'mentally handicapped' people in November 1981. It was seen that inadequacies in community care support led to a cycle of dependence upon institutions. Substantial extra resources were required. The All Wales Working Party was set up and reported in July 1982. The launch of the AWS in March 1983 carried a fund of £26m with it. This fund was to be strategically released over a ten-year period. The main sites for the pilot scheme 'vanguard areas' of the AWS were Rhondda, Arfon and Ynys Mon. The foundation of the Strategy was that it was based on individual need and so a detailed schedule for the whole of Wales would be incompatible with the ethos of the policy. The strategy was based upon the principle of normalisation, that people with learning difficulties had a right to a normal pattern of life within the community. The major responsibility for people with learning difficulties was to fall back on Social Services, but there was expected to be a close liaison with Education and Housing Departments as well as Health Authorities and voluntary groups. The Strategy was unique as it set out a blueprint for participation and representation of people with learning difficulties and their carers in addition to other services. With the thrust of this innovative policy, Social Services were expected to review their day-care provision. This of course highlights similarities with *Valuing People*, which had also called for a review of day services in England (Evans *et al.*, 1994).

In the wake of the pioneering AWS, policymaking in Wales culminated in *Fulfilling the Promises* (2003). This document, similar to those of England and Scotland, covered areas such as person-centred planning and the call for developing self-advocacy. In response to the consultation about *Fulfilling the Promises*, the Joseph Rowntree Foundation (2005) argued that it did not include sufficient recognition of social factors such as discrimination and the barriers people faced. This implied that the policy could have taken more account of the social model of disability. Interestingly this could be linked to the emphasis on normalisation and SRV that was the backdrop to the AWS. There was also comment that not enough effort had been made to really involve people with learning difficulties, rather 'consultation' had been used. However it was noted that the document was far more explicit about the additional need for resources than *Valuing People*, though there was seen to be a risk that funding would be used to consolidate existing resources rather than develop new ones. The Welsh Assembly has given £1.1m to the Advocacy Grant Scheme in the period 2003–07 and around £2m a year for the authorities to implement the policy. The All Wales People First Organisation is nationally active and provides regular conferences and resources to the groups affiliated to it. Therefore England, Scotland and Wales all have a similar policy and funding, albeit limited, to back up advocacy and the voice of the person who uses their services.

Northern Ireland

The governing situation in Northern Ireland is arguably the most complex, rooted in a 200-year history of civil unrest since the 1801 Act of Union. More recently, Northern Ireland has had its own devolved government set up after the Good Friday (Belfast) Agreement in April 1998 (see earlier), which created the Equality and Human Rights Commissions. However, the Northern Ireland Assembly was dissolved in October 2002, bringing back direct rule from Westminster. The Secretary of State and the Northern Ireland Office Ministers have assumed responsibility for the direction and control of the Northern Ireland departments. This leaves questionable the future status of policy and law in Northern Ireland, although it is likely that despite the suspension, future legislation relating to community care will be based in the Department of Health, Social Services and Public Safety (DHSSPS) and either be passed by the Northern Ireland Assembly if it is in place, or, if not, by Westminster.

The Health and Personal Social Services in Northern Ireland are delivered through four Boards, based on Local Authority Districts. These Boards also commission and purchase services for their areas. Since the start of the 1990s, policy developments sought greater equality that involved a range of legislative and policy interventions. Since the mid-1990s, there have also been moves to strengthen anti-discrimination measures. The Belfast Agreement (1998) had a major section on equality and human rights, creating new Commissions. The influence of the Human Rights and Equality Commission focus has reached the central government and provoked change for a similar combination of Commissions for England. For example, the Children's Commissioner for Northern Ireland was the first in the UK. A child with learning difficulties is considered a child in need under the Children Order (NI) 1996. The public authorities in Northern Ireland are charged with constructing equality schemes. These schemes are to be put in place through a process of thorough consultation. The equality agenda will also recognise the differing needs of those with disabilities. However the voluntary and community sectors have found it difficult to cope with the amount of consultation work involved in setting out the equality schemes and policy screening exercises.

The main relevant legislation has been the Mental Health (Northern Ireland) Order 1986. Ideas for improving the management and provision of community care services were set out in the Government paper: *'People First': Community Care in Northern Ireland in the 1990s* (DHSS, NI, 1991). The basic tenets were to encourage independent living away from institutions and the provision of adequate care and support. Most policy and guidance since 1990 has been in line with this aim. The Health and Personal Social Services Trusts in Northern Ireland are overarching, leading to multidisciplinary working. For example, in mental health, learning disability and programmes for the care of elders there has been a tendency for social workers to work alongside medics and paramedics providing a more unified structure of care (Campbell and McColgan, 2002, p. 118).

In 2002, the Department of Health and Social Services issued a *Review of Services for People with Learning Disabilities in Northern Ireland*, which recommitted itself to the underlying principles of independence (DOH, 2002). The Steering Committee for the review included one parent and one person from a self-advocacy group. Similar to the frameworks in England and Scotland, this review so far highlights the need for inclusion by access to mainstream services. The *Review* is said to adopt a transparent and inclusive approach. It emphasises the importance of consulting with users and carers, and aims for the 'full citizenship of all'. However, McConkey notes that in practice, 'it is an unresolved issue as to whether greater participation by people with intellectual disabilities and their carers will provide a major stimulant and contribution to partnership working' (McConkey, 2005, p. 204). Clearly there is much work to be done in including the voices of people with learning difficulties. Indeed, community care in Ireland became private care in residential and nursing homes, many of which are run by former 'mental handicap' nursing staff. The Social Care Institute for Excellence's (SCIE) Board of Trustees and staff visited Northern Ireland in May 2005 to sign a service-level agreement and to strengthen its links with the social care sector. The agreement was to underline the DHSSPS's support of SCIE's work in the provision of good practice guidance and the development of an evidence base of what works in social care.

What is different to England, Wales and Scotland is that there is no separate funding from NI Government for advocacy for people with learning difficulties. Campbell and McColgan (2002) suggest that Northern Ireland, in terms of social policy, is in an ambiguous position because of the profound levels of social and political violence. Over 3000 people have died since 1969 and tens of thousands have suffered injuries of various kinds through institutional, paramilitary and state violence (Fay *et al.*, 1999). Clearly civil unrest has had a marked effect on people's lives, especially on opportunities to develop independently and meet with others at night-time (McConkey, private correspondence, 2002). People First offers a safe forum for members to express their feelings about 'the Troubles'. Currently there is no government funding for independent self-advocacy in Northern Ireland. McConkey (2005, p. 194) points out that government policy has been dominated by the resettlement of people from long-stay hospitals, with a major sub-text being joint working between the NHS and local authority social services.

Conclusion

Osbourne (2003), like McConkey (2005), argues that the Northern Ireland experience has much to offer elsewhere in terms of social policy. The emphasis on human rights and equality overarches the other important aspects of policy for people with learning difficulties and lends itself to a 'social model' approach. That is, people with learning difficulties are viewed as Northern Irish citizens first and foremost. However, there is no evidence that people with learning difficulties have had opportunities to express their own social identities (whether Irish or British). Like so many others in the Province, there is an expectation that children think what their parents think. Equally though, the experience in Northern Ireland has created the development of professional focus on addressing sectarianism and the impact of trauma.

The Welsh and English policies are steeped in the importance of individual needs and person-centred approaches, owing much of their development to the impact of normalisation and SRV theories, which largely shaped them. All the policies have at their core an unstated alliance to these concepts (Race, 1999). Interestingly, the Welsh policy recognises the impact of culture and tradition in different areas and does not attempt to over-centralise service development. Similarly, just as the Scottish institutions led the way in abolishing student top-up fees and establishing free social care, other countries can lead the way in offering policy learning opportunities.

It is apparent that the central government has a lot to learn from policymaking in the other countries of the UK. The view of 'core to periphery' (Hechter, 1975) fails to make this claim. All countries can learn from each other's particular circumstances as each country has different agendas to follow. There is perhaps understandably an irritation on the part of other countries to the approach adopted by the central government in London. Payne and Shardlow point out that the adoption of a national identity for the English has been far more difficult than for other countries: 'the English are frequently constructed as aggressors and imperialists, while other nationalities find pride in self assertion through claims to national identity' (Payne and Shardlow, 2002, p. 21). Interestingly this appears to have been the case for the development of national People First groups, where England has failed to organise a cohesive national network. In summary there are clearly differences between the policies of the four countries and many commonalities. The commonalities appear to centre on advocacy, consultation, person-centred approaches and individualised services.

Part III

The UK Experience in International Context

In Part III, the book explores changes in other Western countries. There were remarkable similarities with the changes in the UK. Common themes are that all the countries were influenced by normalisation; after the Second World War, parents began to join together to fight for improved services; journalists and campaigners exposed poor conditions in resource starved institutions, and these began to close; new ideas, initially focused on better care, later on citizenship, began to influence services; slowly, people began to gain rights to better services; and there were moves to community inclusion. At the same time, change was slow everywhere, and there were still problems with lack of money, poorly-trained staff and patchy implementation.

6
Intellectual Disabilities in the USA: From the Institution to the Community, 1948–2001

James W. Trent

Introduction

From the beginning of the Great Depression in 1929 to the end of the Second World War in 1945, public officials in the United States initiated few changes in policies and services for intellectually disabled people. During the time, several public institutions, like the Rome State School in New York and the Lincoln State School in Illinois, had over 3000 inmates. There were pressures on these and other residential facilities to accept more clientele, but the lack of space prevented all but a small amount of growth. A few states solved the demands for growth by adding new buildings to existing institutions, but most states, without the funds to initiate new projects, did no new building. Some communities, especially in urban areas, had special education classes, but during the Great Depression years, community jobs were scarce for graduates of these classes. For that reason there was pressure on residential institutions to provide care for these unemployed graduates.

With the end of the Second World War and the expansion of American industry in the late 1940s, American officials began building projects that resulted in new residential institutions and additions to the older facilities. In state after state, new institutions were built and quickly filled. The massive and quick growth of these facilities accompanied a change in the social construction of intellectual disabilities. For 20 years, between 1948 and 1968, state public facilities would grow in size and number, and changes in the meaning of intellectual disability would follow changes in its label: from mental deficiency to mental retardation. Only after several converging developments in the late 1960s would the community in the

1970s and 1980s replace the institution to become the locus of care and control for people with intellectual disabilities.

The institution: its critics and its postwar growth

In the United States, the states, not the federal government, operated institutions for intellectually disabled people. After the Second World War, these state facilities had become what Albert Deutsch called the 'shame of the states'. In his 1948 book of the same name, Deutsch had reproduced photographs by Irving Haberman of Letchworth Village, a large institution in New York. The photographs showed wretched conditions. Inmates lay naked on dayroom floors. Vague bodies whirled in repetitive circles of boredom and neglect. Dirty masses huddled together in their own excrement. Once considered one of the nation's most progressive institutions, Letchworth Village had become 'euthanasia through neglect' (Deutsch, 1948).

Letchworth Village represented what had become widespread neglect and abuse in virtually every institution in the United States. Several factors had led to this postwar condition. First, through the years of the Great Depression and the War years that followed, institutions had reached their capacity. Most institutions' group bedrooms could hold no more beds; indeed, many inmates were sleeping in hallways and in day-rooms. Economically distressed states could hardly afford to enlarge existing institutions, and few could build new facilities. In short, state institutions were crowded. Second, during the War years, many of the male attendants and some of the female attendants had joined the armed forces. With the loss of these attendants and with the difficulty of hiring replacements, institutional superintendents during the War years turned to their only source of care-giving: high-functioning inmates. Two decades earlier, superintendents had hoped to place these inmates back into the community. But the Great Depression had made community jobs difficult to find, and the War had made the labour of the high-functioning inmates necessary for institutional care. During the War and postwar years, the high-functioning inmate had become an indispensable part of institutional operations. Third, reports appeared in the press about blatant examples of abuse and neglect in institutions. Most of the brutality came from attendants, but some came from working inmates (Wright, 1947, p. 103).

Overcrowded, without sufficient staff and filled with frequent abuse and neglect, the postwar institution had become what critics called 'a ware-house' or 'a snake pit'. Telling the story of the abusive institution were conscientious objectors, who fulfilled their wartime obligation by serving as attendants in the state facilities. Known as Civilian Public Service (CPS) teams, about 250 men served in 14 institutions around the country. Better educated than most attendants and committed to good care, these men published the *Psychiatric Aid*, a monthly magazine that reported their experiences in state institutions. Their reports described beatings and torture, but, more than anything else, they painted a picture of persistent neglect and sterile routine. To keep their reports before the public, the CPS men in 1946 formed the National Mental Health Foundation. Their reports were not sanguine. Institutions for the mentally deficient had become totally custodial. Virtually no inmates were paroled. High-functioning inmates had become indispensable care-givers to low-functioning inmates. Education and training for residents had stopped. Institutions, the CPS men claimed, could no longer call themselves training schools. Instead they were overcrowded custodial institutions where violence and neglect were commonplace (Angell, 1944, pp. 3–5; Hutchinson, 1946, pp. 241–2; Zahn, 1946a, pp. 5–7; Zahn, 1946b, p. 6; Zahn, 1946c, pp. 4–6).

Aware of the reports of CPS men along with the widely distributed 1948 pamphlet, *Forgotten Children: The Story of Mental Deficiency* (Krause and Stolzfus, 1948), several parents of mentally disabled children began to write about their experiences. This confessional literature began with Pearl S. Buck's 1950 book, *The Child Who Never Grew* (Buck, 1950). First appearing in the popular *Ladies Home Journal* and later excerpted in the even more popular *Readers' Digest* and *Time Magazine*, the book received widespread coverage. Buck told the story of her daughter Carol. Until she was four years old, Carol had appeared normal. But she had walked and talked a little later than most children. In 1924, Buck had Carol evaluated at the Mayo Clinic. There doctors told her that her child was not normal and that the best thing she could do for her daughter was to place her in an institution with children of her own kind. It would be four more years before Buck placed ten-year old Carol at the Vineland Training School in New Jersey. An internationally known author and winner of the Nobel Prize, Buck confessed to being what she called a 'bewildered and ashamed' American parent. Any parent, Buck claimed, even a famous one like herself, could have a mentally deficient child. It was nothing to be ashamed of; parents must not blame themselves. Rather than deny the truth, parents must face reality. Although they might keep their young child at home, parents of mentally deficient children should institutionalize their child by his or her teenage years. Such children needed to be with their own kind. In this environment they would experience happiness (Stirling, 1983).

If Buck's postwar confession represented the stoic, secular response to intellectual disabilities, Dale Evans Rogers' 1953 book, *Angel Unaware*, became its sacred equivalent. Rogers was known to the America public as its favourite cowgirl. With her cowboy husband, Roy Rogers, Dale Evans had appeared in popular motion pictures and was just breaking into television. Her book told the story of her daughter, Robin. Born with Downs' Syndrome in 1950, Robin had died two years later. In heaven, looking down on those she had left behind, Robin told the story of her life and its effect on her family. Rogers assures her readers that her daughter's condition was not the result of heredity. Anyone could have a disabled child. For Rogers, Robin's purpose had a divine intent. A gift from God, a mentally deficient child should be kept at home with her family (Rogers, 1953).

Rogers would give the royalties from her best selling book to the newly organised National Association for Retarded Children (NARC), an organisation made up primarily of parents. In turn, local chapters of the NARC would promote Rogers' book to parents. Although the most prominent examples of the confessional genre, Buck's book and Roger's book were just two of what in the 1950s would become numerous examples of parents who were telling stories about having an intellectually disabled child (Trent, 1994, pp. 220–37). Through the NARC, these parents became, by the end of the decade, one of the most influential human-services lobbies in the nation. From magazine articles to television advertisements, parents got their advice out to the public: mentally retarded children could be helped. And the principal source of this help usually meant the state residential institution. This issue is taken up further in the case of the UK in Chapter 11.

The 1950s and the 1960s marked a time of irony and contradiction in services for people with intellectual disabilities. On the one hand, exposés of the postwar years had uncovered appalling conditions in public institutions. Plagued by overcrowding and inadequate staffing, the public institution through the years of the Great Depression and Second World War had been neglected by public officials and by the public itself. On the other hand, parents of intellectually disabled people were writing about their disabled children. As they spoke out about their children – often under the influence of a family physician who had urged them to put their child in an institution – they made two claims for the public facility: first, ordinary, middle-class families should not be ashamed of placing their disabled child in an institution and, second, public officials must improve and expand existing institutions and must be willing to construct new facilities. Thus, parents in the 1950s became strong advocates for the growth of public residential institutions, an important difference between the aims of parents in the USA and in the UK.

The 1950s and 1960s were a period of enormous growth in public facilities for intellectually disabled people. The postwar Hill–Burton Act provided federal resources for the states in the 1950s to expand existing institutions and to build new ones. In 1963 the Mental Retardation Facilities and Community Mental Health Centers Construction Act would add additional federal funds for institutional growth. Unlike the grand Victorian architectural styles of the nineteenth-century facilities, the postwar institutions revealed contemporary styles:

> Usually single storied, with horizontal windows, plain lines and little if any ornamentation, most newer buildings and additions, nevertheless, kept some familiar features. In most, there were the common tile walls, easy to keep clean and hard to break. In many the floor plans imitated those first devised for the nineteenth-century 'cottage'. Usually a large dayroom separated two or more dormitory rooms, each of which housed two or three dozen residents (as the inmates were generally called by the 1960s). Sometimes a game room and sitting rooms were added to the cottage. Most too had self-contained dining rooms; in some of these there were tables and chairs; in others, a long metal table with round, attached seats that pulled out for sitting and pulled in for easy cleaning. (Trent, 1994, p. 251)

Not only would the institutions of the 1950s and 1960s be different from their predecessors, they would also differ from earlier institutions by their population. Between 1946 and 1967, the population of facilities for intellectually disabled people in the US increased from 116,828 to 193,188, an increase of 65 per cent and nearly twice the rate of increase in the general American population. Besides this population increase, the institutions of the 1960s would appear different to those of their predecessors in another way. From the last two decades of the nineteenth century through the 1940s, many of the inmates admitted to the public institutions were so-called defective delinquents. These juvenile delinquents – usually teenagers and young adults – were placed in institutions for the intellectually disabled to keep them out of trouble. In institutions, these delinquents often worked on the institution's farm or provided care to more disabled inmates. In the 1950s and 1960s more severely disabled children and adults would replace the 'defective delinquent'. During these decades the shift in populations meant that the public institution would have a greater number of severely disabled residents without the free labour provided by the higher-functioning juvenile delinquents. As such, institutions found themselves having to hire additional staff. Although federal resources supported the construction of new institutions and the additions to old institutions, the states continued to be responsible for funding the day-to-day upkeep and staffing of the institutions. By the end of the 1960s these costs would become prohibitive for many states, and with under-funding, reports of institutional abuse and neglect would reappear.

The demise of the institution

As the number and populations of institutions grew in the 1950s and 1960s, lingering memories of the 'snake pit' facilities of previous decades remained. Indeed, in the midst of institutional growth, social and economic factors would build to discredit the residential institution as the principal source of services for intellectually disabled people. The first of these factors could be seen in Eunice Kennedy Shriver's 1962 article in the *Saturday Evening Post* (Shriver, 1962). While John Kennedy was in the White House, the article acknowledged that the Kennedy family had a retarded sister. Besides this acknowledgment, Shriver stressed that retarded children and adults could be helped. Also, under favourable conditions, Shriver claimed, retarded adults could live in the community. Around the same time, other articles appeared in the popular press that stressed a similar theme: retarded children could be helped and the institution was not the inevitable outcome for retarded people (Kollings, 1962; Strait, 1962; Woodring, 1962; Oettinger, 1963).

As parents of intellectually disabled children and adults, led by the Kennedy family, began to add the community as a place for their children, so too did a new group of critics of the institution begin to appear. First and most prominent among this group was Erving Goffman with *Asylums* (1961). Funded by the National Institute of Mental Health, Goffman had spent a year in St Elizabeth's Hospital, a mental health facility in Washington, DC. In this institution, Goffman observed the daily routines and interactions of patients and staff. From his observations, he argued that the mental health facility operated as a 'total institution'. By total institution, Goffman meant that mental health patients were deprived of their individuality, and the institution caused patients to react in 'deviant' manners and behaviours. 'Labeled deviants, institutionalized patients only reacted with more hostility, thereby confirming the label' (Trent, 1994, p. 254). Soon the labels became so much a part of the patients' identities that coercion and shame became unnecessary as the total institution became routinised in day-to-day institutional life. In short, the patient absorbed the label. Goffman insisted that mental illness, and, by extension, mental retardation, were not essential; rather, they were socially constructed labels (Goffman, 1961).

Also appearing in 1961 were two other books critical of the mental health system. In Thomas Szasz's *The Myth of Mental Illness* and Gerald Caplan's *An Approach to Community Mental Health*, the question of the reality of mental illness was raised. In different ways, each book claimed that the labels created by professionals usually reflected the convenience of the labeler. As such mental illness was a myth. Also, institutions were holding facilities for the myth; in a sense, they were merely myth-maintaining facilities. In any case, the institution was beyond improvement. The best policy would be the elimination of the institution (Caplan, 1961; Szasz, 1961).

Approaching the public institution from different, but nevertheless, damning perspectives were studies published in the early 1960s by the California sociologist, Robert Edgerton. Like Goffman, Edgerton observed inmates; unlike Goffman, he observed intellectually disabled inmates. What he saw in the institution was a place 'constitut[ing] a staggering visual, auditory, and olfactory assault on the presupposedly invariant character of the natural normal world of everyday life' (McAndrew and Edgerton, 1964, p. 314). Later in the decade, Burton Blatt and Fred Kaplan published their collection of photographs and narrative, *Christmas in Purgatory* (1966). Reproduced the following year in the popular *Look* magazine, the photographic essay created the greatest amount of mail in the history of the magazine. Like the exposés of the late 1940s, Blatt and Mangel's *Look* article pictured the institution as a place of 'neglect, filth, and pervasive boredom, all characteristics of a "Christmas in Purgatory" ' (Blatt and Mangel, 1967).

Along with these professional writings that doubted the assumptions of mental health services and of the public institution, the early and mid-1960s also produced popular criticisms of the institution. In 1962 Ken Kesey published his book, *One Flew Over the Cuckoo's Nest*, and in 1967 Philippe de Broca's film, 'King of Hearts', appeared. Both the novel and the film suggested that the sane, not the insane, were the oppressors. 'The mad [knew] more about sharing, cooperation, and joy than [did] the rest of warring, manipulative, greedy, and power-driven humanity' (Trent, 1994, p. 255). The institution was no more than a place for exploitation and cruelty (Kesey, 1962). Within these professional and popular criticisms of the institution, parents and professionals in several of the states – New York, California, Alabama, Illinois, Pennsylvania and Washington – began in the mid- and late 1960s and early 1970s to raise more doubts about the place of the public institution in providing care for intellectually disabled people.

In September 1965, Robert F. Kennedy, a United States senator from New York, strongly criticised two of the state's largest facilities, the Willowbrook and Rome State Schools. As a senator, Kennedy had little influence over the state government in Albany, but given the traditional interest of the Kennedy family in mental retardation, Kennedy's criticism gained the attention of the press and the state's public officials. For nearly a decade, the governor of the state, Nelson A. Rockefeller, had focused his attention and a large proportion of the state's budget on the Albany Mall Project, an extensive construction project of public buildings. In the process, state residential institutions had received reduced funding. Kennedy addressed a joint session of the New York legislature. What he portrayed was not a pleasant picture. Institutionalised mentally retarded people, Kennedy claimed, were denied access to education and were 'deprived of their civil liberties by being forced to live amidst brutality and human excrement and intestinal disease' (Rivera, 1972, pp. 52–6; 'Where Toys Are Locked Away', 1965).

Under attack in New York, the residential institution also found itself under attack at the opposite end of the country. In California, Governor Ronald W. Reagan, in January 1967, had ordered all state agencies to eliminate ten per cent of what he characterised as 'fat' from their budgets. From state mental health hospitals and state mental retardation facilities, he had specifically demanded that officials eliminate $17m from their annual budgets. Reagan reasoned that this cut would eliminate 3700 state jobs, close 14 state outpatient clinics and begin a course of community-based care. Reagan insisted that it was time for communities to take care of their own 'mental patients'. When protests came from state mental health advocates, Reagan reacted by claiming that public facilities were the 'biggest hotel chain in the state' (Kerby, 1967).

Later that year, Niels Bank-Mikkelsen, the director of the Danish national services for mental retardation, observed conditions in the Sonoma State Hospital, a large California institution for retarded people. Although Reagan's budget reductions had not yet fully taken place, Bank-Mikkelsen found appalling conditions in the institution. He informed a reporter: 'I couldn't believe my eyes. It was worse than any institution I have seen in visits to a dozen foreign countries ... In our country, we would not be allowed to treat cattle like that' ('Question of Priorities', 1967). What he reported were wards of naked adults sleeping on tiled floors often in their own excrement. Most inmates were heavily medicated. It was not uncommon for drugged residents to move randomly about in a pharmacological daze. Screams and shouts only added to the surreal atmosphere. In reaction to Bank-Mikkelsen's comments, the California Commissioner of Health and Welfare insisted that the state's treatment of the retarded was 'the most advanced in the nation'. Bank-Mikkelsen feared his claim might be true.

Just as Governors Rockefeller and Reagan were reducing state support for institutions in New York and California, so too did Governor George Wallace of Alabama begin cutting back on funding for public institutions. Hoping to honour his recently deceased wife, and former governor of Alabama, Lurleen Wallace, George Wallace planned to make the University of Alabama's Medical School in Birmingham one of best facilities of its kind in the nation. To concentrate public funding there, Wallace proposed what, by all accounts, was inadequate funding for state residential institutions (Cavalier and McCarver, 1981; Lerman, 1982, pp. 159–64).

In Illinois, as had been the case in New York, California and Alabama, Governor Richard Ogilvie proposed laying off paid staff at the Lincoln and Dixon State Schools, the two largest residential institutions in the state. Already hurting from the loss of 'fewer working students', or high-functioning inmates who had already been discharged, employees of the two institutions worried about the care of low-functioning residents. Protests from parents and elected officials delayed the lay off for a time, but inmate care remained a concern (Watson, 1970a, 1970b).

In the fall of 1968, Gunnar Dybwad, a consultant for the Pennsylvania Association for Retarded Children (PARC), reported to the membership that the only solution to the terrible conditions in the state's public institutions was to launch a lawsuit against the state. Parents feared that such a suit would jeopardise their relationships with state officials. At the PARC's 1969 annual meeting in the following spring, John Haggarty, the Association's Executive Director, shared information from his inspection of the state's public mental retardation facilities. During his presentation, he showed a slide of a boy at the Pennhurst State School. The boy had died of burns under questionable circumstances. The slide had the effect that Haggarty hoped it would; the PARC sued the state before the year was out.[1]

Back in Alabama, state employees were also considering a lawsuit against the state. Still concerned over the dismissal of professional and care-giving staff at state institutions, employees feared new layoffs and reduced funding. In 1970 the employees had attorneys initiate a class-action suit against the Alabama Department of Mental Health.

The Pennhurst suit in Pennsylvania and *Wyatt v. Stickney* in Alabama represented important legal events in what would become a decade of litigations:

> By 1973, from legal actions to prohibit involuntary servitude in mental retardation institutions (which had the effect of depriving institutions of their traditional and cheapest source of labor) to suits guaranteeing equal educational opportunities in public schools, advocates for [intellectually disabled] citizens were heading in the direction of closing public institutions and eliminating self-contained special public schools and classes. (Trent, 1994, p. 257)

In 1972 New York institutions were once again in the public light. Geraldo Rivera, then a young and little-known investigative reporter, visited New York's two largest mental retardation facilities: Willowbrook State School on Long Island and Letchworth Village in upstate New York. He brought with him television cameras. In February 1972, Rivera's exposé, 'Willowbrook: The Last Disgrace', aired on prime time television to 2.5m viewers. Around the same time, several New York newspapers carried the stories of Willowbrook and Letchworth. What television viewers saw and newspaper readers read were conditions that were not unlike the death camps of Nazi Germany. All the inmates contracted hepatitis within six months of entering the institutions. Most of the severely disabled inmates were not clothed. As such, they lay naked in their beds or on dayroom floors. It was not unusual for them to be lying in their own faeces. The smells in both institutions were insufferable. Rivera learned that between 1968 and 1970, New York state officials had reduced Willowbrook's staff of 3383 by 912. Most of these employees were direct patient-care workers. In addition to these reductions, Willowbrook was scheduled to lose an additional 300 employees. With exposés like Rivera's that continued to surface in the late 1960s and early 1970s, parents and advocates seemed to echo Rivera's claim, 'We've Got to Close the Goddamned Place Down' (Rivera, 1972).

Just as the institution came under scrutiny so too did the segregated Special School and special class. Community-funded schools had for decades provided education to intellectually disabled children, but these schools and classes were almost always segregated from so-called normal schools and normal classes. Several federal programmes – Project Head Start and the Elementary and Secondary Education Act (ESEA), for example – had provided funding that supplemented state and local funding. School programmes for intellectually disabled children were included in this legislation. Despite the additional funding, programmes remained segregated, and parents and educators in the early 1970s began to question them.

Their questioning was supported by academics who were beginning to challenge the very notion of mental retardation. In these critiques mental retardation was not an essential reality; rather, it was a label ascribed by authorities to certain children who were members of racial minorities and from lower classes. Jane Mercer's 1972 article, 'IQ: The Lethal Label', which appeared in the popular magazine, *Psychology Today*, was an example of the challenges to the labelling of public school children. According to Mercer, some school children became mentally retarded because school authorities had ascribed the mentally retarded label to them. Their 'mental retardation' was less related to their mental capacity than to their race and class. Placed in segregated special education programmes, these children behaved in ways that fulfilled the ascribed label. After the children left school and returned home, they showed that they could behave quite well in day-to-day neighbourhood and community life. They were what Mercer called 'six-hour retarded children'. Labeled retarded for six hours while in school, they functioned quite normally after school. They were only 'retarded' at school (Mercer, 1972).

Into communities

In the early 1970s, two groups began to advocate for moving intellectually disabled people from public residential institutions and from segregated schools and classes to communities and to integrated classes in community-funded schools. The first group contained state and local officials impatient to reduce costs for large public institutions, and the second group were advocates eager to close what they saw as cruel residential facilities and ill-conceived special education programmes. They were strange bedfellows – cost cutters and civil libertarians. The mix of their motives has continued to trouble services for intellectually disabled citizens to the present.

Deinstitutionalisation, beginning in the early and mid-1970s, was made possible by federal legislation and funding. Changes to the federal health care programme for the poor, Medicaid, and the enactment of the federal programme for the poor, Supplemental Security Income (SSI), allowed for the transfer of institutionalised intellectually disabled people from public institutions to community-based facilities. For the first time in American history, the federal government rather than state governments would fund services for intellectually disabled people. In 1973 the United States Congress passed the Education for All Handicapped Children Act (PL 94-142). Among other things, the Act mandated that community-funded schools provide education for *all* children, including those with disabilities. The federal legislation had been modelled on a 1971 Washington state law that had guaranteed public education for all the state's children (Schwartzenberg, 2005). For many intellectually disabled children, the federal legislation had meant schooling in regular schools and in classes with non-disabled children (Marcus, 2005).

In the 1970s through the 2000s, states across the country depopulated public institutions. In Illinois, for example, the Lincoln State School and Colony dropped its population from over 5000 in the 1960s to 383 residents in 2000. In 2002, the state closed the institution. Letchworth Village in New York went from 4000 residents in the 1960s to 630 in 1990. In 1996 the facility shut its doors transforming much of its extensive grounds into a golf course. Since 1970 nearly 50 public institutions in the United States have closed. Some have become institutions of an alternative incarceration – usually prisons. Among these closed facilities are the older institutions, but several of the institutions built after the early 1960s have also closed. Although states have maintained some institutions, most of the facilities are small, usually not having more than a few hundred residents. In most cases, these residents have severe or profound intellectual disabilities (Braddock *et al.*, 1990; Gehlbach, 2001, p. 3).

Having left the public institution, where have intellectually disabled people gone in communities? Many have gone to small, home-like group homes, or so-called Intermediate Care Facilities (ICFs), and some are living independently or with minimal assistance from, for example, a social worker. Some, like my friend, Carl (not his real name), in the mid-1970s left a large state institution to join a group home with four other intellectually disabled men, who were assisted by a live-in 'house coach'. After a few years of adapting to the community, Carl left the group home to live independently. He learned to drive and eventually purchased a car. A few years ago, he married. Like the rest of us, he has the normal problems and joys of day-to-day living, but his adjustment to the community has gone well.

Although there are many examples like that of Carl, there are also examples of the reinstitutionalisation of intellectually disabled people in the community. Indeed, many people left the public institution only to live in large group facilities of over 15 beds. Most of these facilities are nursing homes (Braddock, 1987; Braddock *et al.*, 1990). In these facilities, residents often experience boredom and neglect, not unlike what they experienced in the large institution.

At the beginning of the twenty-first century, intellectually disabled people who live independently or semi-independently in American communities face two major problems. The first is employment. Where the state and national economies are relatively strong, intellectually disabled people find jobs. Yet, many of these people lack health care insurance, and, for that reason, are economically vulnerable. At the same time, during economic downturns, intellectually disabled people are often the first to lose their jobs (Zaslow, 2005). The second problem concerns the eligibility for Medicaid and SSI that most disabled people are dependent upon. Since the early 1980s during the Reagan administration, these programmes have received lower federal funding. More recently, the administration of George Bush has convinced the US Congress to reduce payments to both programmes to pay, in part, for the war in Iraq. By the early twenty-first century, then, the community has become 'beloved' for many intellectually disabled people – for those with jobs, with families and with friends. They have what Robert Putnam (2000) calls 'social capital'. Yet, for many others – for those without employment, without adequate public assistance, without community resources for services or for those who have been reinstitutionalised in nursing facilities – the community has become, without 'social capital', a 'lonely crowd'.

Note

1. Interview between the author and Gunnar Dybwad, transcribed 12–14 June 1990.

7
The Development of Community Services for People with Learning Disabilities in Norway and Sweden

Jan Tøssebro

Introduction

Internationally, Scandinavian policies for people with learning disabilities are probably best known for the principle of normalisation. Nirje's formulations in a North American book in 1969 are widely known. However, the idea had already been around for some time. It existed as a sensitising concept in the early 1960s, and a Danish law text from 1959 stated as a goal that people with learning disabilities should have the opportunity to *live a life as close to normal as possible*. The resettlement from institutions to community services in the Nordic countries can be regarded as a gradual commitment to, and implementation of, the principle of normalisation. However, the concept continues to be a sensitising concept rather than one with a fixed and specific meaning, and the meaning has changed over the years. 'As close to normal as possible' is very different today compared with 1960. The service developments should however also be related to the concept of social justice – a reaction to the living conditions of people with learning disabilities and a commitment to the welfare state ideal that society should have a responsibility for providing acceptable living conditions to all citizens.

From a distance, the Scandinavian countries may appear similar to one another. Seen from the countries themselves, however, one is more inclined to stress the differences. The history of community services has similarities, but also differences, and a description of their evolution would entail too much detail if attention was paid to all differences. This chapter is thus mainly on Norway and Sweden, with only occasional references to the other countries. These two countries are among the few that closed all institutions in the late 1990s. The history of community care cannot be separated from the history of deinstitutionalisation, partly because it grew as an alternative to institutions, but also because the ideology was more explicit that the institution was not wanted, than about what the community alternative should be. This chapter will thus be as much about deinstitutionalisation as the coming of community care. It will be organised in four sections; the emergence of alternatives to institutions (mainly the 1960s); the early ideological discourse; the early deinstitutionalisation (1970s and 1980s); and the full scale replacement of long-stay institutions (1990s).

Emerging new services in the golden age of institutions

The 1950s and 1960s were the golden age of institutions in all Scandinavian countries, but also the years when the first signs of new ideas and services appeared. All countries expanded their institution-based services in these decades. In Sweden and Denmark, the number of residents peaked in 1970–71, with about 1.7 persons per 1000 inhabitants living in residential institutions for people with learning disabilities. This is a somewhat higher rate than in the UK and USA (Ericsson and Mansell, 1996), though the peaking of numbers is almost simultaneous. In Norway, Finland and Iceland the increase in number of residents levelled off around 1970 with about 1.3 persons per 1000 inhabitants. The peak was, however, a bit later, in 1976, and took the shape of a plateau (1970–90) rather than a peak (Tøssebro *et al.*, 1996).

In these years, the institutions dominated the service system. The service ideal was large institutions. (Norway and Sweden actually also set up a number of smaller institutions, but this was for practical reasons, not because people questioned the benefits of large facilities.) The only real alternative was that the family cared for the individuals with learning disabilities with little or no public support. Gradually, however, the first signs of changing patterns emerged, both with regard to services and ideological climate. It is not clear which was first, but service development definitely started before the new ideology grew strong. The early service development was not about resettlement from institutions, but about providing a broader range of options. Day services, non-residential schools and sheltered workshops were provided for people living with their families. These new services were sometimes at a Day Centre, but even total institutions developed day services for non-residents ('day patients'). In Danish institutions for instance, services for non-residents hardly existed in 1950, whereas in 1960 the institutions had admitted more than 2000 day users (20 per cent of all users).

The new developments appeared first in Sweden. In the 1940s, a Public Committee argued that generic services to a larger extent should serve people with disabilities, and a 1954 Act (on education and care for people with learning disabilities) triggered new service development. This law argued the case for locally-provided special education and sheltered workshops (Ericsson, 2002). Similar developments took place some years later in Norway, and in the beginning, practical and economic arguments were more important than ideology. It was argued that the costs of residential schools were three times those of day schools, where children lived with their parents. Thus, one could provide services for three times more people for the same money. The year 1959 actually became a sharp demarcation line. Before 1959, all Special Schools for children with learning disabilities were residential and mostly located in rural areas, whereas all established after 1959 were in towns or cities, and children lived with their families. Day services (schools, sheltered workshops) were most important among the new services, but even 'sheltered accommodation' emerged in these years. In Sweden the first units were set up in the 1950s, whereas the development started in the 1960s in Norway. Such accommodation was, however, a small part of the service system until the 1970s in both countries.

The emerging new services were for children and adults with mild and moderate learning disabilities, not people with extensive service needs. And even though the focus of this book is mainly adults, it cannot be overlooked that services for children played a vital role at the 'turning point'. In the 1960s, a new division of labour between families and public services was born. Developments in Norway illuminate this. Around 1960, the development of non-residential Special Schools was based on economic considerations, but within a few years the arguments changed. In 1967 the Government, in a White Paper to the Parliament, claimed that the family could provide better care than any institution (White Paper 88, 1966–67, p. 20) and that the role of the public should be to support families so that children with disabilities could grow up in a normal family environment. This was in part a result of a heated debate on residential Special Schools. They were subject to severe criticisms regarding living conditions and abuse; on national TV a famous film director compared them to concentration camps (1967). The debate led to an investigation by the Ombudsman, who concluded that even though criticisms were exaggerated, residential schools were not a place to spend a childhood (1967). A childhood as normal as possible became the new guideline. Day services, respite care and economic support gradually developed, and the number of children in institutions and residential Special Schools peaked. From the early 1970s, even children with severe and profound learning disabilities were provided with alternative services, after being granted the right to education, in 1967 in Sweden, and in 1970–75 in Norway.

Thus, children came to be the *avant garde* with respect to the development of alternative services, and particularly with regard to people with severe disabilities. The change took the shape of a new division of labour between the public and the families – from the earlier 'either family or total care' to the current 'both family and public support'. However, it was also the first strong official commitment that institutionalisation was undesirable.

Changing ideologies

The new types of services were about creating more options, not to replace long-stay institutions. As the momentum grew stronger, so did the ideological critique of total and segregated services. The idea of normalisation was important. However, a careful reading of the discussions in the 1960s suggests a debate with many strands. The bottom line appears to be that the earlier 'solution' to the problem of learning disability, the institutions, gradually came to be seen as *the* problem.

Roughly speaking, there were three main ideological arguments. The first came to be related to the purpose of institutions, but at the outset it was about the return of a long-gone optimism regarding the potential of proper treatment to make a difference to people's potential. All people learn, so the argument went, provided the environment and treatment are adequate. Subsequently, this neo-optimism led to dissatisfaction with the custodial role of institutions. In both Norway and Sweden, reformist child psychiatrists came to play a vital role, and ideas about adequate nursing changed. At the largest Norwegian institution, the ideal nurse of the 1950s was said to be one that efficiently kept the unit clean (Hellan, 1992), but twenty-five years later it was the teaching of communications skills to people with challenging behaviour. Among professionals, the conception of the purpose of institutions changed from custody to rehabilitation. Active care, teaching and a stimulating environment became the issues, and discharge to a less restrictive environment the goal.

The ambition thus became changing institutions into treatment centres. The case for more staff, better qualified staff, a more stimulating environment and a more active care was argued. It did not initially lead to a plea for the closure of institutions. However, some child psychiatrists did make a link with labelling theory. According to this perspective, society's reactions to deviant behaviour tend to reinforce this behaviour. Prisons are criminal schools rather than correction centres. Institutions for people with learning disabilities provide fewer stimuli and learning opportunities than other environments and thus tend to be learning disabling. The experiments of Tizard (1964), for instance, in the UK (outlined in Chapter 1) were referred to as evidence (Rasmussen, 1962). The main implication of the new purpose was however not deinstitutionalisation, but reformation – the normalised institution.

The second type of critique was about living conditions. Not that living conditions deteriorated during the 1950s, on the contrary, but in the early 1960s expectations changed. A bed was no longer sufficient. The Scandinavian countries began to see themselves as welfare states. It became a part of the political self-image that society provided acceptable living conditions for all citizens. This self-image fostered new expectations, and also a new wave of social criticisms, particularly from radical social science. The argument was that this self-image did not reflect the harsh realities experienced by some groups of people. Thus, both new expectations and a more fertile ground for social criticism came into being, manifesting itself in media scandals. In Norway an *ad hoc* action group with several celebrities among its members argued that segregation in institutions was a way of concealing the appalling living conditions that society provided for people with learning disabilities (Skouen, 1969).

Lastly, segregation in itself came to be seen as more problematic. Segregation has hardly ever been a valued measure, but with the influence from the Civil Rights movement in the USA – the 1954 Supreme Court ruling that 'separate is *not* equal' – the stigmatising effect was seen more clearly. In Norway, critics of institutions in the mid-1960s pointed to the similarities between segregation in institutions and apartheid. It was argued that segregation was a violation of civil rights. Politically speaking, the defence of current policies became problematic. When the ambition is to be a welfare state and a society for all, how could it be justified to plan and organise segregation of groups of people – and place them at a stigmatising site? The reply came: only when alternatives cannot be provided.

It is mere speculation, but it appears as if a change in the focal point took place in the 1960s, and all the three arguments outlined above are interconnected. During the years of expanding institution-based care, the main focus was on families. The point was to make it possible for the rest of the family to take care of itself and live a normal life. But gradually, and definitely from the mid-1960s, the individuals with learning disabilities themselves became the focal point – with regard to individual development, living conditions and stigmatisation. Thus, the quality of services came to be much more important.

As a consequence of these criticisms and ideological developments, strategies to change the pattern of care were put on the political agenda in both Sweden and Norway. Sweden revised its Service Act in 1967 and introduced a couple of changes in order to avoid unneeded institutionalisation. The preferred option for children became special classes at local schools; all children were granted the legal right to education (including those that earlier were seen as 'uneducable'), and children who could not live with their families were be accommodated in small 'pupils homes'. For adults, group homes and supported independent living programmes became the preferred options. The institution came to be seen as a last resort. Day programmes were developed irrespective of whether people were living in or outside institutions. However, some people were seen as 'needing' this type of services, and adults with severe disability were still expected to live in institutions.

In Norway, a Public Committee identified three goals for service development – integration, improved living conditions and the stimulation of adaptive behaviour (NOU 1973, no. 25). The goals were interrelated. Improved living conditions in institutions was not only a goal in itself, but also a means to provide a more stimulating environment for learning adaptive skills, which subsequently made discharge (integration) possible. The strategy was dual. First, institutions became the least favoured option – a last resort. Day programmes and respite care were to make it possible for children to grow up with their family, and adults with lesser service needs were to be provided with services outside institutions. The second strategy was to improve, decentralise and normalise the undesired option – to improve institutions and make them more desirable. They should become more home-like, smaller, move into communities and provide more day programmes and cultural activities.

The ideology in the two countries appears fairly similar, and the development from about 1970 was in some respects similar, but there was one important difference. In Sweden there was a real 'take-off' of alternatives to institutions. In Norway this only happened for children.

Deinstitutionalisation phase one: community care and normalised institutions

The first years of deinstitutionalisation in Scandinavia were characterised by four developments: children gradually disappeared from institutions and residential schools; day time options were created for adults and adolescents living with their family; institutions were normalised; and adults with lesser needs were resettled in the community. The resettlement of adults into the community mainly applied to Sweden and Denmark until the late 1980s (Tøssebro *et al.*, 1996).

It may seem odd to call the reformation of institutions deinstitutionalisation. However, both at the time it occurred and with hindsight, institution improvement appears as a part of the normalisation movement. It was not only about living conditions and an environment for learning adaptive skills but also about changing the unwanted option in the desired direction. Institutions were to become a less typical version of the species, 'total institution'. This was seen as the only possible development in services for adults with substantial service needs. And improvements definitely took place. Norway can serve as an illustration (Tøssebro, 1992).

Even though Norway had had both small and large facilities since the early 1950s, the priority changed in favour of small ones in the late 1960s and early 1970s. The new facilities were usually set up in towns and cities, population centres (small and large) rather than in rural areas. The proportion of the institutionalised population that was living in small facilities grew from 35 to 55 per cent in the 1970s and 1980s; the mean size of large facilities declined from 225 to 140 residents; and the mean size of all institutions from 59 to 23. Nearly all institutions were renovated and many larger facilities were reconstructed according to the image of a village. The mean number per ward or living unit dropped from 23 in 1971 to 6.5 in 1989, and by 1989 nearly all (96 per cent) had their own bedroom (12 per cent in 1971). Staffing levels are perhaps the most illuminating measure. The total staff: resident ratio started to increase around 1960 and sharply from 1970. In 1960 there were about 0.4 staff per resident, in 1971, 0.63 and in 1989, 1.81 – more than four times the ratio in the 1950s and early 1960s. Houses became more home-like, interaction with the community more common, and the rhythm of the day and year more similar to everyday life. In many respects there was a quantum leap according to the ideal of *living a life as close to normal as possible*. But the facilities continued to be institutions run and licensed according to the Act on hospitals, and with little or no use of generic services.

In Sweden a similar development took place, but in addition a number of people moved out of institutions. The number of 'beds' in institutions declined by 15 per cent during the 1970s. The pace increased in the 1980s, as seen in Figure 1, which also compares with Norway. Note that it was not until 1980 that Sweden had fewer people in institutions than Norway.

There are no obvious explanations for the diverging patterns between Norway and Sweden. The ideology appears not to be very different, and

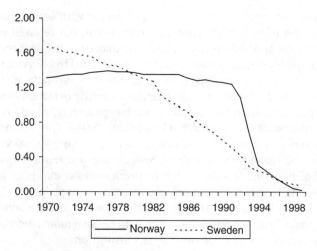

Figure 1 People in Institutions for People with Learning Disabilities in Norway and Sweden per 1000 inhabitants, 1970–99.
Source: Tideman and Tøssebro, 2002.

neither were the policy guidelines. One explanation may be that more people with lesser service needs were initially institutionalised in Sweden (more people were in institutions in Sweden, but it is unclear whether this was because Sweden institutionalised more people with lesser service needs or because Norway had longer waiting lists). The administrative structure of the service system probably played a role. In both countries institutions were run by the county (regional) authorities. In Sweden these authorities were also responsible for community services, whereas in Norway, community alternatives were supposed to be organised and funded by the local (municipal) authorities. This produced a financial incentive for not acting among local authorities in Norway. If they did not provide services, they could hope that the counties 'solved' the problem by admitting people to institutions. The Public Committee that proposed a full dismantling of the institution-based system in Norway in 1985 (NOU, 1985, no. 34) argued that the shared/divided responsibility had been an efficient barrier to the development of community services, and the problems linked to the shared/divided responsibility were also one reason for implementing deinstitutionalisation in one grand move.

The community accommodation that slowly emerged from the late 1950s was basically of two types. First, people living semi-independently – either in small units spread over a housing area, in boarding-houses or in blocks with small units for all sorts of people with accommodation needs. Some users had virtually no service needs, but received generic social services and had irregular help (for instance finding daytime occupation). Others had moderate service needs provided by a service unit in the area. Second, people living in group homes – typically about five people – shared a house or large apartment (mostly detached houses of villa type) and with in-house staffing. Each person usually had his or her own bedroom (Ericsson, 2002; Grunewald, 2004). The first type of community accommodation was available both in Norway and Sweden, whereas the second was mainly in Sweden (but existed in Norway as well). Furthermore, few people left institutions for community accommodation in Norway; it was more often an option for people leaving the family home. Larger hostels with 20–25 residents were not common in Scandinavia. That is, such units existed and became more common, but were generally seen as small, normalised institutions.

In addition to community accommodation, day services expanded during the 1960s, 1970s and 1980s – mainly schools and sheltered workshops. Such workshops could be within institution grounds, admitting both people living in the institution and outside ('day patients'). The workshops could also be centres operating independently of the institutions, and even these units admitted both people living inside and outside the institutions. In Sweden such centres served about 7000 people in 1980 and 14,000 ten years later (Grunewald, 2004). In Norway they expanded from about 1000 in 1970 to 3150 in 1989 (Tøssebro, 1992). Note that Norway's population is about half of Sweden's.

In the middle of the 1980s, the normalisation movement entered a new phase. In Sweden, the number of people with community accommodation outnumbered those in institutions (Grunewald, 2004), and political initiatives were taken to speed up the process. Community living was no longer only for people with lesser service needs. In Norway, the number in community accommodation fell far short of those in institutions, at about 20 per cent (Tøssebro, 1992), but impatience regarding the changes seen as desirable was growing – and this impatience did not distinguish between mild and severe disability. (Initially they planned to keep institutions for people with challenging behaviour and autism, but this was changed during the process.)

Deinstitutionalisation phase two: replacing institutions

Based on the work of a Public Committee (SOU, 1981, no. 26), the Swedish Parliament revised the legislation on services for people with learning disabilities in 1985. The Public Committee argued that institutions had a negative impact on the personal development of residents, were an obstacle to a good life, and that housing was an individual right that should be made available to all (Ericsson, 2002). According to the 1985 Act, new admissions to institutions were no longer permitted unless a crisis existed. Furthermore, all people living in institutions were granted the right to an annual assessment to determine whether the person could be transferred to more normalised service options (Grunewald, 2004). The institutions were in fact no longer seen as a service option and were supposed to be phased out. However, no final deadline was set.

In Norway, a Public Committee proposed full dismantling of institutions in 1985 (NOU, 1985, no. 34), based on similar arguments to those in Sweden, adding that 'institutions are humanly, socially and culturally unacceptable' (p. 12). It also argued that earlier 'soft' policy guidelines and recommendations had been proven to fail and that stronger measures were needed. It thus recommended both a fixed timetable and the abolition of the earlier shared/divided responsibility for services. From a specified date, local authorities were to be solely responsible for services. By and large, the recommendations were unanimously approved by the Norwegian Parliament, and in 1988 mandated by law, with an implementation timetable from 1991 to 1995.

The decline in numbers of people in institutions is shown in Figure 1. About 80 per cent of the residents in Norwegian institutions were resettled in the community by 1994, and 60 per cent moved in a big wave in 1991 and 1992. It took a bit more time to resettle the last individuals, but by 2000 the era of institutions had come to an end. In Sweden, the gradual reduction of people in institutions continued. The Swedish Parliament therefore enacted mandatory closure in 1997, and by the deadline in year 2000, only 80 individuals (compared to 13,000 in the peak year 1970) remained (Tideman, 2004). Currently, all institutions are closed in both countries.

It is not straightforward to explain why the policy on institutions changed in the 1980s, from 'unwanted but necessary' to simply 'unwanted'. Some points are however worth noting. One aspect is that the undesirable option came to be seen as even more undesirable; the voices backing the arguments evolving in the 1960s grew stronger. Another more practical issue is staffing: it was obviously more feasible to resettle people with severe service needs with the staff ratio of the late 1980s as compared to that of the 1960s. A third point is the changes in the general service system; community care had in general gained a much more important role in welfare services during the 1970s and 80s. This applies to people with all kinds of disability, old people with medical needs and also children with extensive service needs, for instance with multiple disabilities. When these children could be served in co-operation with families, why were institutions needed for adults? Furthermore, the whole image of disability changed, from a medical or health issue to a question of equality and participation. The social justice part of the arguments of the 1960s had become the main argument, and with respect to realisation of social justice, any 'qualification' based on service needs was unjustified. And last but not least, the parents' Societies were strongly advocating full dismantling of institutions. The last point is worth a word or two. It is true that the parents' Societies were very critical of institutions and advocated their dissolution. However, when it came to implementation, it turned out that families did not agree. Many feared that the closure of the one service they knew would end in disaster. Opposition grew which is one reason why implementation took longer than planned. However, after resettlement, most changed their minds. About three out of four deemed the new services better (Tøssebro, 1997; Ericsson, 2002; Tøssebro and Lundeby, 2006). Internationally, it seems to be a fairly general pattern that families fear institution closure, but change their minds subsequently (Larsson and Lakin, 1991).

One argument against closing all institutions was that some people had very complex service needs, due to, for example, medical needs or challenging behaviour. The Public Committee that proposed total dismantling in Norway argued that in reality most of these services were provided or supervised by outside experts on a part-time basis, even in the institutions. Thus, closure of institutions did not necessarily make much difference. However, to address the issue, both countries set up regional 'expert' teams that are supposed to support community services on an outpatient basis in cases with complex service needs.

The main structure of the community services in Norway and Sweden was established during the reform years in the 1990s. Local authorities are responsible for services in both countries, and the public itself is the main service provider. Most people tend to live in group homes consisting of three to five units. Each person in the group home has his/her own unit with bedroom, sitting room, bathroom and kitchen, usually around 50m². In addition, there tend to be communal rooms and staff rooms. Others live semi-independently. This can be in singular units in an apartment block, or several units scattered around a housing project area and with one unit serving as staff unit, service centre and communal area. Semi-independent living appears to be more common in Sweden than in Norway, whereas purpose-built houses are more common in Norway. Most people have day activities, but rarely regular jobs. They tend to be at Day Centres or sheltered workshops (Tideman and Tøssebro, 2002).

In general, evaluations have tended to suggest that the resettlement led to improved living conditions for people with learning disabilities (Tideman, 2000; Tøssebro and Lundeby, 2002; Ericsson, 2002), but also that far from all problems were solved. The gap between ideals and reality is widening. There is, for instance, a concern about micro-institutionalisation, about integration being merely physical and that people with learning disabilities continue to live in a world apart. Space does not permit addressing these issues here, but some examples from Norway illuminate the point (Tøssebro and Lundeby, 2002; Tøssebro, 2005). The daytime activity of most people with learning disabilities is either at a Day Centre for people with learning disabilities (56 per cent) or at a sheltered workshop (31 per cent). Very few are at a regular workplace and only 14 per cent have a colleague without disabilities (management and supervisors excluded); that is, a world apart. Furthermore, the number of former institution residents that frequently take part in leisure activities organised for the general public has not increased after resettlement. Modern neighbourhoods are rarely characterised by tight social networks, but most people socialise with neighbours. Thus, in the general Norwegian living conditions survey, 73 per cent replied that they knew at least one neighbour well enough to pay occasional visits. Among people with learning disabilities, the corresponding figure was 28 per cent. It is also worth noting that about a quarter of the new units actually are on or near the grounds of the closed institutions and that four out of ten live in a neighbourhood with more care facilities (mostly more group homes but even larger facilities). This does not mean that the reforms did not make any difference – they did. But even though institutions are closed, a milder version of segregation continues to exist, and there are definite possibilities to move further down the road in order to make community services less institution-like.

Conclusion

During the 1990s, community care replaced institutions in Norway and Sweden, even for people with severe learning disabilities. The unwanted but necessary option of the 1970s was no longer perceived as needed.

The current service system was established during the 1990s, and few changes have taken place since. There are however some recent developments. More people live semi-independently (Ringsby Jansson, 2002; Tøssebro and Lundeby, 2002), but this occurs alongside a trend to group more people together. These new and larger arrangements tend to house people with service needs, but not necessarily for the same reason. Thus, a house could accommodate elderly people, people with physical impairments, mental illness and learning disabilities. Thus, in some municipalities, the challenge today may be of a defensive nature, to avoid a backward movement – to larger facilities and more groups of people with service needs. There is one more positive development that should be noted. Both in Sweden and Norway, community care today serves more people than the institutions ever did. In Norway 2.4 persons with learning disabilities per 1000 inhabitants received community services in 2000 (11,500 people, cf Circular I-19/2000), whereas the corresponding figure in Sweden was 2.1 in 2004.[1] Although one should be cautious about direct comparison with the figures from institutions, both are significantly higher than the 1.3–1.7 rates of 1970.

Note

1. The figure is based on the number receiving 'accommodation with support' according to the Act on special services (LSS). *Source*: website of the National Board on Health and Welfare, February 2006. http://www.socialstyrelsen.se/ Publicerat/2005/8793/Sammanfattning2005-44-5.htm

8
The Evolution of Community Living in Canada: Ontario, 1945–2005

Tim Stainton

Introduction

This chapter considers the evolution of community care using Ontario, Canada's largest province, as a case study. It covers the period from the Second World War to 2001. As community care is a provincial responsibility, no national lens is possible, hence the use of a case study, though its experience in many ways mirrors that of other provinces. As in the United Kingdom, the War years saw increasing concern for public welfare in Canada and the beginnings of the welfare state. The federal Government issued in 1943 the Marsh report (Armitage, 1975, pp. 216–17). This report, similar to and influenced by the Beveridge Report, recommended a comprehensive set of income security measures. This was followed in the 1950s with a series of 'categoric programmes' which provided for means tested benefits cost-shared between the federal Government and the provinces. This cost-sharing approach became characteristic of Canadian programmes and allowed the federal Government to spur welfare reform despite health and social services being constitutionally under provincial jurisdiction.

From 1872 there had been a slow but steady increase in numbers of people with learning disabilities identified in provincial institutions. Economic and ideological constraints had limited institutional development; in 1930, Canada had institutional provision for less than 2000 people, with fewer than 200 special classes in schools (Kirkpatrick Strong, 1930, p. 190). A lessening of financial constraints in the immediate postwar period, coupled with serious overcrowding and huge waiting lists, engendered a programme of institutional expansion. Overall,

Ontario's institution population grew until 1964, eventually reaching 6424 (Simmons, 1982). Spurred on by the new cost-sharing mechanisms (Williams, 1984) in 1952 Ontario introduced a means tested benefit for 'any person totally and permanently disabled' between the ages of 18 and 65 and not living in an institution. One effect was to reduce the stigma associated with government benefits because it included middle and upper income families. Williams notes that 'the mentally retarded who had been secluded since childhood as a family secret, their existence scarcely noted by the neighborhood, were now brought forward to qualify for government aid, and thereafter they enjoyed a brighter life' (1984, p. 77). One need not share Williams' optimism to accept the benefit of bringing families 'out of the closet'. Indeed perhaps the single most important event of the 1950s, as elsewhere, was the advent of the organised parents' movement.

The parents' movement and the growth of education

As in the UK, the parents' movement began with a letter to the editor (Anglin and Braaten, 1978, pp. 6–7; Simmons, 1982, pp. 149–50).[1] It came from a carer who was frustrated with the lack of support for children who, having IQs of less than 50, did not qualify for any educational or training programme. The letter spawned a follow-up by another parent asking concerned individuals to attend a meeting in a Toronto church. Seventy people responded and aims were defined, concerned primarily with educational opportunities. A delegation met the Minister of Education on 9 November 1948. This marked the beginning of parent involvement in policy-making. The parents organised themselves, first into local councils and in 1953 into the Ontario Association for Retarded Children (OARC) (Anglin and Braaten, 1978, pp. 6–7; Simmons, 1982, pp. 150–1). The first 'experimental school' for children with IQs under 50 was started in 1947 supported by a grant from the provincial Government. There was also a 'pilot programme' in Toronto financed by the federal Government begun in 1949. There had been a few special classes prior to this, explicitly for people with a mental age equivalent to school age. These classes were also used as a 'clearing house' to identify those who should be transferred to institutional care. Henceforth many parents were reluctant to have their children enrolled in them (Simmons, 1982, pp. 90–1).

In September 1952, the Parents' Council opened the first auxiliary school. In June 1953, the Government agreed to provide $25 per month for each pupil. These auxiliary schools would remain the primary source of education until 1969, when the Ministry of Education took over responsibility (Anglin and Braaten, 1978, pp. 7–10; Simmons, 1982, pp. 151–2). The Government was reluctant to accept responsibility for community programmes, but was ready to subsidise the voluntary sector. This is in part explained by Ontario's 'residualist' or minimal state involvement approach to social welfare. The Canadian welfare state was driven not so much by social democratic ideals as by a liberal ideology (Moscovitch and Drover, 1987). The early decision to subsidise the voluntary sector rather than undertake direct service provision at either the local or provincial level is perhaps the most significant divergence between the UK and Ontario.

The OARC grew rapidly. By 1962, there were 85 local associations (Anglin and Braaten, 1978, p. 30). The Canadian Association for Retarded Children held its first conference in 1958 (Anglin and Braaten, 1978), and with its inception came the establishment of the tripartite structure which continues to operate. Local bodies focused on service development and delivery; the provincial bodies focused on policy and programme development, and the national organisation, given the muted influence of federal policy on people with learning disabilities, was free to focus on advocacy from a position of relative autonomy. While the relationship between the levels has been strained at times, this separation of roles and powers allowed for a unique combination of influence and capacity not seen elsewhere.

Voices for change: the early years of community care policy

Towards the end of the 1950s, in the midst of a major institution building programme, voices for change began to be heard. Dr Matthew Dymond, who took over as Minister of Health in 1958, began to articulate a new policy for mental retardation. In February 1959 he outlined his proposals, the most important of which was the establishment of the Children's Psychiatric Research Institute in London, Ontario (Zarfas, 1976, p. 268; Simmons, 1982, pp. 163–4). The 1960s were a period of unprecedented interest in learning disability. This was inspired by both the critique of institutions and renewed interest in the US spawned by President Kennedy's Committee on Mental Retardation. There was also a public exposé of conditions in the institutions. The 1960s were ushered in by a dramatic report in Canada's largest newspaper on conditions in Orillia, Ontario's largest institution (Berton, 1959). This, coupled with pressure from the OARC, forced the Government to begin to rethink its policy. Two reports in 1963 pointed to the need for expansion of community services (Roberts, 1963; Simmons, 1982, pp. 170–8). While accepting the general thrust of these reports, the Government had no intention of taking on full responsibility for community services. The institution remained the key government-operated and funded service (Simmons, 1982, p. 170). Dymond presented a Blueprint for Mental Retardation Programming in Ontario on 7 June 1965.

While there was little that was new or radical in this document it represents one of the first attempts to bring coherence to Government policy. Perhaps the most important development was the creation of the Mental Retardation Services Branch within the Ministry of Health to co-ordinate services. It also established an Inter-Departmental Committee on Mental Retardation Policy on which the Ontario Association for the Mentally Retarded (OAMR), formerly OARC, was represented (Zarfas, 1976, p. 270; Anglin and Braaten, 1978, p. 39; Simmons, 1982, p. 184). Two key pieces of legislation followed, the Homes for Retarded Persons Act 1966 (HRP) and the Vocational Rehabilitation Act 1966 (VRA). The HRP provided part capital grants and funding for approved operating costs of approved charitable organisations. The VRA provided part capital costs operating grants to vocational programmes, primarily sheltered workshops (Zarfas, 1976, p. 270; Simmons, 1982, p. 185). The major take-up was under the VRA, and by 1970 there were 84 sheltered workshops as compared to only eight residences, four of which were operated by local associations (Simmons, 1982, p. 185).

While we noted earlier that numbers in institutions peaked in 1964, this figure is misleading. The reduction was largely due to the introduction of the Homes for Special Care Programme (HSC). This was aimed at getting people who 'could not benefit from active treatment' out of institutions and into more 'home like community settings'. They were placed in private facilities, usually nursing homes, where costs were low and care custodial the best (Simmons, 1982). Presented as a programme of community service provision, it was primarily a means of reducing costs through accessing newly available cost-sharing monies under the Canada Assistance Plan (CAP) (Simmons, 1982, pp. 186–8). The HSC programme remained a continuing source of scandal into the 1980s (OACL 1987a, b; Ontario, ComSoc, 1987). This was the only widespread use of private services and a consistent source of scandal. This contrasts with the UK where private services did not play a significant role until the 1990s.

Yet while an enormous amount of rhetoric emanated from the Government about the need to reorient mental retardation policy away from big custodial institutions towards some form of community care, at no time did it provide either the leadership or sufficient funds to establish adequate comprehensive community facilities or services for mentally retarded people. Almost every major change that occurred was the result of outside pressure, from OAMR, from the press or from opposition attacks in the legislature (Simmons, 1982, p. 165). While the rhetoric was more impressive than the reality, the 1960s saw the establishment of subsidising voluntary groups to provide community-based services. But as in the UK, scandal was the tipping point for significant movement.

The Williston Report: indicting the past, charting the future

In 1971, two tragedies forced a review. On 18 February, Jean-Marie Martel, recently discharged from Rideau Regional Centre, was found on a country road with gangrenous fingertips caused by frostbite. Martel had been placed in a local farm, a common practice where local farmers looking for cheap labour requested workers from institutions. Newspaper reports catalogued abuse and neglect (Williston, 1971, pp. 13–19). Then, on 5 March, police found Fredrick Elijah Sanderson, a 19 year old on leave from Rideau Regional Centre, hanging from barn rafters, having committed suicide. Like Martel, he had been sent out to work on a farm (Williston, 1971, pp. 8–13). The Minister of Health asked Walter B. Williston, a Toronto lawyer, to investigate. He gave Williston a wide brief, asking him for 'some clear direction as to both government and public responsibility for such persons'. He stated 'as we move into this whole area of human rights we immediately get involved in fundamental legal issues, particularly those concerning the civil rights of citizens, whether or not they are retarded' (Williston, 1971, pp. 3–4).

Williston's report is one of the most remarkable in the history of learning disabilities in Ontario. He argued that problems concerning mentally retarded persons could not be viewed in isolation; civilised society should provide all children with the opportunity of developing to their optimum potential; and the furnishing of the basic necessities and support to enable people to function in society should be recognised as basic human rights (Williston, 1971, pp. 4–5). Williston called for large institutions to be phased out as quickly as possible, noting problems of overcrowding, custodialism, antiquated buildings and isolation. He also made an economic case, as institutions inhibited rehabilitation and made it more difficult for people to adjust to the community when released. Williston concluded that: 'a century of failure and inhumanity in the large multi-purpose residential hospitals for the retarded should, in itself, be enough to warn of the inherent weakness in the system and inspire us to look for some better solution' (Williston, 1971, pp. 67–8). This is reminiscent of Peter Townsend's comment on British institutions 'the disturbing conclusion has to be faced, that the wrong system of care has been developed' (Townsend, 1969, p. xxvii). Both indicate an early acceptance that the fault was with the institutions themselves, not in their operation.

Williston recommended that the institutional population be reduced to 40 per cent of current capacity. He recognised that institutions would have a role to play 'for some years to come', but that this would be along-side efforts to support parents through a range of services and benefits to keep their children at home (Williston, 1971, pp. 71–3). In other words, a 'comprehensive community service system' would have to be provided. He reinforced the use of local voluntary groups such as the OAMR, argu-ing that the Government should not build or run accommodation, work-shops or leisure facilities in the community, but fund the voluntary groups that were providing these services (Williston, 1971, p. 98). The idea of community services being funded by government but provided by voluntary groups recognises government's responsibility to ensure sup-port; it also recognizes the weakness of large bureaucratic public services and the strength of local concern which can be achieved by voluntary bodies (Simmons, 1982, pp. 225–7, 243). This is a key point of contrast with the UK, where the state was both funder and provider.

Ideology and economics

Williston's recommendations were not accepted across the board, though over the next few years many of his ideas came to the fore. Other significant forces influenced the pace and direction of change. One was the concept of normalisation, which began to receive wide attention at the end of the 1960s (Nirje, 1969). Two key figures in normalisation philosophy were in Ontario in 1971. Bengt Nirje was the coordinator of training at the Ministry of Health. He was one of the originators of normalisation; his very presence suggests a favourable disposition to normalisation. More radical, and ultimately more influential, was Wolf Wolfensberger, who became visiting scholar at the National Institute for Mental Retardation in Toronto in 1971. One cannot discount the force of Wolfensberger's personality in assessing the impact he had on the general climate in Ontario and elsewhere (Wolfensberger, 1972; Simmons, 1982, pp. 195–7). His uncompromising value-based approach amounted to an ideology, where one was either 'for or against' his ideas. Wolfensberger also questioned the role of the voluntary sector as provider of services (Simmons, 1982, p. 196; Wolfensberger, 1984). Nirje and Wolfensberger's influence was critical to the reforms which followed Williston.

The initial response to Williston was to scale down the largest facilities by transferring people to smaller institutions closer to their home (Simmons, 1982, pp. 199–200). There was, however, at this time a general reorganisation of the provincial Government in order to improve efficiency. Robert Welch was appointed Minister of Social Development Policy; he was somewhat sympathetic to learning disability issues (Simmons, 1982, pp. 201–2). Welch appointed a task force which in April 1973 produced the Green Paper *Community Living for the Mentally Retarded: A New Policy Focus* (Ontario, Provincial Secretariat for Social Development, 1973). This spelt out for the first time a commitment to the idea of normalisation and a reorientation from institutions to community-based services. It rejected the idea of a Ministry for the Handicapped on the basis that this would be 'segregating handicapped citizens from other citizens in Ontario'. It favoured transferring the institutions to the Ministry of Community and Social Services (ComSoc) (Anglin and Braaten, 1978, pp. 65–6; Simmons, 1982, pp. 203–7).

This was not an ideological decision. The transfer from Health to ComSoc made the province eligible for 50 per cent cost-sharing 'with the stroke of a pen' (Anglin and Braaten, 1978, pp. 66–7; Simmons, 1982, pp. 207–8).[2] The Developmental Services Act (DSA) came into effect in April 1974 giving ComSoc responsibility for all mental retardation facilities. It also provided an umbrella under which ComSoc could institute programmes beyond those authorised under the HRP or the VRA. What had been a relatively small Ministry with some 2000 staff ballooned to 12,000, the majority based in institutions (Williams, 1984, p. 127). The result was paradoxical given the goal was to reorient services to the community, because it gave the Ministry an institution-based staff and budget.

The community service division was initially committed to the implementation of community living. While the 1970s generally was a time of restraint within ComSoc, mental retardation services were exempted from this (Williams, 1984, p. 128). This allowed some innovations, but progress was slow. By 1976, the initial optimism was waning and the consensus on the direction of policy both internally and externally was weakening. The bureaucracy became increasingly filled with career civil servants with no particular commitment to community living and perhaps a greater concern for economy (Simmons, 1982, p. 244). The sheer number of institutional staff ensured that they increasingly dominated the ComSoc bureaucracy. Unlike in the UK, direct care staff did not transfer to the community from the institutions. Community-based staff were generally trained through the Community College system or were untrained staff hired directly into community agencies. Other factors which slowed deinstitutionalisation include the reduced influence of the OAMR, community resistance to group homes and increasingly active resistance by the Ontario Public Service Employees Union to institutional closures (Simmons, 1982, pp. 240, 223–4).

The Government's major tactic was the by now well-worn solution of building smaller institutions. The large institutions began to respond to the threat to their existence, both by claiming 'normalizing environments' within, and by proposing themselves as 'centres of expertise', a concept supported by ComSoc through the promotion of 'resource centres' (Simmons, 1982, pp. 222–3; Coalition Against Institutions As Community Resource Centres, 1986). By 1980, there had been no significant reduction in the numbers of people in institutions and there had been a net increase in their number. There was, however, a significant development of sheltered workshops and to a lesser degree of community residential places (Simmons, 1982), as well as the Adult Protective Service Worker programme which combined advocacy and case management and was a prelude to future directions.

The failure to make significant reduction in institutional populations mirrors the UK. In addition to this was the difficulty in developing community services and indeed knowing what services to develop. There were, however, positive steps and lessons being learnt which encouraged success in the 1980s. The ComServ project of CAMR sought to develop local experimental and demonstration projects based on normalisation aimed at creating a comprehensive community-based service system. While the outcomes were mixed, it served to focus thinking on the 'how to' of community services (Lord, 1985; Roeher, 1976). There was also the development of the PASS evaluation system and citizen advocacy projects, as well as the beginnings of the self-advocacy movement in Ontario. These developments set the stage for the actual phasing out of institutions in the 1980s.

Institutional closures and programme innovation

The 1980s began with several hopeful changes. The long neglected Homes for Special Care Program was reformed and the Government announced $29m for assessment and developmental training programmes (Simmons, 1982, pp. 235–9). But it took seven years and several scandals to get the children and young adults out of the nursing homes and homes for special care. In 1980, Bill 82 was passed which guaranteed the right of all children to special education services and programmes without payment by parents. The Government instituted two significant community programmes, the Special Services at Home Program and the Assistive Devices Program. These programmes were expanded in 1990 to include adults and were the first direct funded programmes in the province (Ontario, ComSoc, 1987, pp. 5–8; Ontario Office of Disabled Persons, 1988). A new five-year plan called for the closure of six institutions and the reduction of a seventh, affecting around 1000 people.[3] From leaked internal documents, it was clear that the motivation was cost savings and the plan was widely criticised (McWhorter and Kappel, 1984).[4] Much of the criticism came when, after two closures, 100 of the 150 people moved to other institutions. The later closures were more successful and five of the six centres closed with reductions to the others (Ontario, ComSoc, 1987, p. 8).[5] The plan was typical of deinstitutionalisation plans of the 1980s with those considered 'high functioning' moving out, strong economic motivations and little in the way of individualised planning or coordination. It was more an exercise in service rationalisation than any positive development of community services. It was, however, a beginning and demonstrated the feasibility of closing large facilities in a reasonably short space of time. By 1985, the number of people in the community had risen to over 4500 with an increase in expenditure on community-based services from $10m in 1974–75 to $181m in 1985–86. Some 33,000 people were receiving Government support by 1987. However, residents in institutions outnumbered those in community residential services (Ontario, ComSoc, 1987, pp. 5–8).

Emerging citizenship

From 1985, a new Liberal Government unleashed a torrent of policy reviews, including the Social Assistance Review Committee; the less high-profile Review of Advocacy for Vulnerable Adults; and the Advisory Committee on Substitute Decision Making for Mentally Incapable Persons (Ontario, ComSoc, 1988).[6] While the content is important, what is more significant are the concerns they reflect and the debate they engendered. The range of consumer and advocacy groups which appeared before these reviews testified to the changing landscape. Where previously the OAMR had been the only group concerned with learning disability, it was now but one voice in a large crowd. The

Advocacy review received over 30 submissions from groups with a direct interest, including from Ontario People First which had formed earlier in the decade.

The nature of these reviews reflects a significant shift in the relationship between the state and marginalised groups. The traditional paternalistic concern with 'how many residential spaces' and 'how best to help these unfortunates' is supplanted by concern for enhancing autonomy and rights (Ontario, ComSoc, 1988, pp. 107–12; Torjman, 1988, pp. 101–5). This denotes a shift from the traditional, residualist/paternalist approach to a perspective grounded in notions of rights.[7] It needs to be set in the context of the 1982 Canada Act which included the Canadian Charter of Rights and Freedoms, the first to explicitly include learning disability.[8] It has had a significant impact on the legal equality of people with learning disabilities. Two cases are of particular note – first, the 'Eve' case which ruled that a non-therapeutic sterilisation without consent could not be performed despite the wishes of a legal guardian, her mother and second, a case that involved the right to vote under the Canada Elections Act. The Act excluded people whose 'liberty was restrained' or whose property was under the control of a trustee because of 'mental disease'. These sections were declared in contravention of the Charter giving large numbers the right to vote for the first time.[9]

In May 1987, ComSoc for the first time committed to the complete elimination of institutional care. This, however, was tempered by several factors. The reduction targets for the seven year period were significantly less ambitious than those advocated by the OAMR, now the Ontario Association for Community Living (OACL) and many other groups (OACL, 1987a, 1987b). No fixed timetable was given for the complete closure of institutional facilities in the Government document. While the document clearly indicated that it aimed to continue the use of community voluntary agencies to provide community services, it proposed two additional approaches termed 'divestment and diversification'(Ontario, ComSoc, 1987, p. 23). Diversification was intended to placate the unions but it met with strong opposition by the OACL and others concerned over the transfer of institutional norms and practices to the community (OACL, nd). There was, however, a clear commitment to expand community services, particularly those services which provided flexibility, integration with generic services, choice and portability (Ontario, ComSoc, 1987, p. 15). It called for joint planning with consumers and service providers, noting the need to increase individualised support, and the development of models such as case management to achieve this (Ontario, ComSoc, 1987, pp. 28–9).

Conclusion

Ontario continued its faltering progress towards community living through the next decade and a half. Some innovative programmes developed and progress was made in closing the institutions, though at the time of writing this had still not been achieved with a target date of 2007. British Columbia by comparison had closed all its facilities by 1996. The 1970s represented the high watermark of optimism and radical vision, a vision that became mired in bureaucracy and economic rationality. On a broader front, there was an increasing concern with rights and citizenship, though its expression in terms of appropriate supports remains work in progress. The community living movement also changed, with a growing self-advocacy movement challenging the system. In many ways, Ontario mirrored the UK and other countries in the move to community living. The unique character of Ontario and other Canadian jurisdictions with split government funding and community organisation delivery spawned many innovations and an active advocacy movement. In the end, however, the failure of vision and commitment on the part of the Government authorities, plus the reluctance of well-entrenched service providers, has delayed both the return to community and the building of inclusive communities.

Notes

1. *Toronto Daily Star*, 29 September 1948.
2. Interview between the author and David McCoy, 27 September 1990.
3. Statement by the Honourable Frank Drea, Minister of Community and Social Services, 28 October 1982.
4. Ontario Public Service Union, *Services To The Developmentally Handicapped: A Five Year Plan For Disaster* (Toronto, 1983).
5. 'Plan to Shut Retarded Centres Called Attempt to Save Money', *Globe and Mail*, 12 September 1984; 'Liberating the Retarded', *Toronto Star*, 3–5 January 1983.
6. Attorney General of Ontario, *You've Got a Friend: A Review Of Advocacy in Ontario* (Toronto, 1987); Submission to the Ontario Ministers of Health, Attorney General and Community and Social Services and Minster Responsible for the Office of Senior Citizen's Affairs, *Final Report of the Committee on Substitute Decision Making* (Toronto, 1987).
7. Submission, *Final Report of the Committee on Substitute Decision Making*, p. 49.
8. Canada, *The Canada Act*, 1982, S.15 (2).
9. Federal Court of Canada, Trial Division, T-1787-88.

9
The Mirror Cracked: Care in the Community in Victoria, Australia

Kelley Johnson

Introduction

> And moving thru' a mirror clear
> That hangs before her all the year,
> Shadows of the world appear ...
> The mirror cracked from side to side.
>
> Tennyson, 1832

Like the Lady of Shalott, many people with learning difficulties in Australia, early last century, saw life as a reflection viewed through institutional windows. Then in the 1980s, the mirror cracked. People with learning difficulties began to leave institutions, others were not admitted and more began to live their lives in the wider community. Unlike the Lady of Shalott this did not mean they were doomed, although it has to be acknowledged that the dreams and aspirations of those involved in the deinstitutionalisation movement have not been fully realised. This chapter begins with one person's narrative to illustrate some of the changes that have moved some people with learning difficulties from being mirror gazers on life to being more active participants. It also examines the limits of these changes and how they have reflected in microcosm wider themes in our society. The chapter focuses on changes occurring in one Australian state (Victoria), because it led the way with the reforms that occurred for people with learning difficulties. However many of the reforms and changes instituted in Victoria were later reflected in changes in other states.

Kirsten's narrative[1]

'Inside the day room, Kirsten stands by the glass door leading to the dining room. She gazes out through the panes. She holds her hands on either side of her face and whimpers quietly. In one of her hands she holds a plastic mug which she rarely relinquishes' (Johnson, 1998, p. 27). Kirsten is a tall russet haired woman who was 39 years old when I met her in the locked Unit of an institution for people with learning difficulties. She had lived in the locked Unit for 13 of the 19 years she had spent in the institution. Kirsten did not use speech, found it difficult to eat and needed a lot of support with toileting and dressing. She lived in the locked Unit with 20 other women of varying ages. Kirsten was timid and shy. If I stood quietly beside her for a time she would reach out a hand, briefly stroke mine, then withdraw hastily. She spent her days moving around the walls of the Unit, or standing gazing out of the windows. I learnt that often she sought the places where the sun was shining and would stand for hours in a patch of sunlight. She seemed afraid of the other women and was sometimes attacked by Brigid who would rush at her and pull her hair. Kirsten would stand weeping until staff took Brigid away. She had been admitted to the locked Unit ostensibly because of challenging behaviour. At times she would stand and scream, short sharp bursts of sound which broke her usual silence. Her stomach was constantly distended and though medical examinations had been inconclusive, it seemed to cause her pain and discomfort. A warm bath seemed to ease the pain and stop her screams for a time.

Kirsten showed no other 'challenging behaviour' although staff reports recorded that she had 'dirty habits' which seemed to consist of masturbation. In order to prevent this, her hands had been tied behind her back in earlier times. She had been admitted to the locked Unit because she had been found in a man's room in an open Unit, and staff thought she was vulnerable to sexual abuse. After admission to the locked Unit, she was given contraceptive pills.

Kirsten had lived with her parents until she was 20 years old. She was one of nine children, two others of whom had disabilities. Kirsten had contracted an illness in infancy leaving her with severe learning difficulties. Doctors told her mother that she 'would never be any good' and should go to an institution. However her parents decided that she should remain part of the family. Her mother was her main carer. The task was not easy. She did not have any support in caring for her family, and Kirsten did not attend any community-based services but was always at home. Her mother commented:

Some nights she wouldn't want to go to bed and some nights I'd have to sit up till three or four o'clock in the morning until she decided to go to bed. Because if she didn't want to go to bed she'd keep on getting

out, well even if you lock doors you just can't go to bed and leave a
child like that wandering around the house ... I mean she could fall in
the dark and lie there bleeding while you're sleeping and not knowing:
and you had to stay up. (Johnson, 1998, p. 51)

Social work reports on the family revealed that Kirsten was a loved and
included member of her family. However, eventually her mother could
not care for her any longer and she went to live at Hilltop.

Although the institution was a long way from her family home, for
some time Kirsten's parents took expensive public transport to visit her
regularly. Her father could not bear to visit her after he found her one day
with her hands tied behind her back, but her mother recalled visiting and
eating tubs of ice-cream with her in the institution grounds. As her
mother became older and more frail, she found the journey too difficult
and had not seen her daughter for six years at the time of my research.

When the Government decided to close Hilltop, her mother and
sisters visited her to discuss with staff where she would live after the
institution closed. Kirsten was incredibly excited at seeing her family,
rushing in circles around the table where they sat and stopping by her
mother to touch her briefly. Her mother was anxious about the institution's closure. She was afraid that the promised community support
might fail and she would be forced to care again for her daughter. At the
same time she thought that Kirsten would be happier and more content
in the community. The institution closed and Kirsten moved to a suburb
closer to where her mother lived. She now lives in a house with four
other people with learning difficulties, supported on a 24 hour basis by
staff. She attends a day programme for some hours each day.

Kirsten's life reflects in microcosm some of the enormous changes in
policy relating to people with learning difficulties in Australia. All of
these changes had implications for 'community care'. This chapter
explores some of the changes that have occurred during Kirsten's lifetime.
It focuses particularly on changes in relation to deinstitutionalisation,
advocacy and the development of rights legislation.

1940s–70s: life as a reflection

Kirsten was born at a time when institutional care was still the primary
focus of service delivery for people with learning disabilities. The doctor's advice that Kirsten should go to an institution is reflected in other
accounts by parents: 'they [the doctors] then said: "You must make up
your own minds, of course, but in our opinion you should put him in

the Kew Cottages [an institution for people with intellectual disabilities] and forget him. Never visit him again" ' (Temby, 2005, p. 138). Some parents took the doctors' advice. Kirsten's mother did not. Her experience of raising a child with learning difficulties highlights the lack of community-based support that was then available. There was little direct support for families caring for children with learning difficulties and access to day care depended on parental knowledge and individual advocacy. When Kirsten's mother was unable to care for her, the institution was the only alternative offered.

Once Kirsten entered the institution there was an assumption (implied at least) that she would be there for life and that her experience of the community would be limited to her view from the windows and infrequent excursions or holidays which remained institutionalised events (Judge and van Brummelen, 2002). Because of concerns about her sexuality and gender, Kirsten was prevented for a long time from participation in the limited occupational therapy available to people living at the institution. There were no activities within the locked Unit in which Kirsten could be involved. Her removal from the community gradually also removed her from her parents. Her 19 years of life there were restricted in large part to the locked room in which she spent her days.

The 1980s: the mirror cracks

The decision to close the institution in which Kirsten lived was part of a radical change in the discourses about people with learning difficulties which occurred in Victoria in the 1980s. There was a movement from constituting people with learning difficulties as patients, or as sick, to a discourse which framed them as citizens with the right to live a life as close as possible to other citizens.[2] In part this shift was due to the impact of writers from the United States (Wolfensberger, 1975) to repeated scandals and concerns about institutions in the state (Office of the Public Advocate, 1990; Wallace, 1991). Also significant were economic pressures related to the cost of institutional care and broader rights discourses which in Australia were framed around Aboriginal land rights and the rights of women. The new thrust of Government policies was to acknowledge that people with learning difficulties had rights and that these should be safeguarded through a range of advocacy and accountability mechanisms. In Victoria, the shift was revolutionary in its range and effects. It was reflected in changes in the law, the development of advocacy services and the movement from institutions to supported housing and community services for people with learning difficulties.

Government was not only to provide opportunities for people to exercise their rights to their full potential, but it was going to be made accountable for doing so. The following examples illustrate this change.

In 1986, the Intellectually Disabled Persons' Services Act was passed in Victoria and was one of the few Acts in the world to focus particularly on people with learning difficulties. It reflected a profound change in attitude to people with learning difficulties. The Act identified them as citizens with rights. The first of its set of 14 principles stated that 'intellectually disabled persons have the same right as other members of the community to services which support a reasonable quality of life'.[3] In the Act, there was a focus on the importance of maximising physical and social integration, utilising generic rather than specialist services, ensuring that one organisation did not have total control over an individual's life, and encouraging consumer participation. Following the passing of the Act, a ten-year plan was developed by consultants employed by the State Government (Neilson Associates, 1987a, b; 1988; Naufal, 1989). Over a two year period an intensive review of services for people with learning difficulties was documented and a State-wide consultation was held with advocacy groups, parents, and government and non-government agencies. The result of this was a ten-year plan which was highly critical of institutional living for people with intellectual disabilities and which argued strongly for a transition from institutional life into community-based services. The ten-year plan was translated by the Government into a three-year plan which came into effect in 1989 (Community Services Victoria, 1989). This Plan set objectives for services over the following three years. It involved an increased commitment by Government to Disability Services, of $26.5m, to develop services which would increase community services such as employment, day programmes and residential services.

Target numbers were established for new services and there was a focus on the needs of people with intellectual disabilities living with older parents and people residing in institutions. The State Plan did not meet all of its objectives. Because of increasing financial problems, the State Government did not implement a second three-year plan but concentrated in 1992 on the closure of a large institution for people with intellectual disabilities, moving 220 people into the community and transferring the rest to other institutions. Both the Neilson Report and the State Plan used the language of rights to establish a rationale for their objectives. There was an air of optimism in both steps which was reflected in the promised injections of Government funding into the intellectual disability area and in the development of new services.

Since the early 1970s, parent advocacy groups in Victoria had been a strong voice arguing for better quality of life for people with intellectual disabilities in the state (Temby, 2005). During the 1980s, this voice was given added impetus by Government recognition of the importance of advocacy in all its forms. As part of the rights discourse, the Guardianship and Administration Board Act was passed to establish agencies which would act as safeguards for people's rights.[4] This Act established an Office of the Public Advocate and a Guardianship and Administration Board to advocate for people with disabilities, to safeguard their rights as citizens and to provide assistance in the form of guardians and administrators for those people who found it difficult to make life decisions.

The Office of the Public Advocate was a strong voice in arguing for systemic change in disability services and policies. It produced an annual report which was tabled in Parliament, and it also produced a report from community visitors who were able to enter, without warning, all institutions around the state to check on the quality of services and on abuse of rights. These reports were highly critical of institutional life for people with learning difficulties and were an important ingredient in the movement towards deinstitutionalisation (Community Visitors, 1990; Office of the Public Advocate, 1990). The Public Advocate's Office urged Government accountability for the services it provided and its reports were couched within a rights discourse. Two self advocacy groups and a number of other advocacy organisations representing families and people with learning difficulties received funding from the Government. These groups carried out research, publicised issues affecting their constituents and had a place on Government policymaking bodies.

During the 1980s, there was an increasing emphasis on the need for people with learning difficulties to live in the community. Governments made commitments to closing institutions and gradually some of the largest institutions were closed. There was general agreement that large institutions were not fit places for people to live, and a number of reports from the Office of the Public Advocate and other Government-commissioned reports supported this movement (Office of the Public Advocate, 1990; Wallace, 1991).

Kirsten's departure from the institution reflected the changes in policy during the 1980s. The institution in which she lived was closed in part because of strong advocacy which exposed the poor quality of life, isolation and abuse of people living there. Legislation provided a guide to the provision of stronger community care services and Government was committed to the provision of community housing and day services. However Kirsten's living arrangements were organised within narrow limits based largely on funding issues. A community residential Unit of four to five people and a day programme or activities were provided, but there was little individual choice about where, with whom, or how Kirsten would live in the community.

From reflection to a new reality: 1990–2000

During the 1990s, there were wider changes in the community that affected the lives of people with learning difficulties directly. In Victoria a Conservative government won office, and managerial and strongly individualistic discourses gained dominance. The effects of this change are reflected in the following examples.

The Intellectually Disabled Person's Act was retained. A review of the Act emphasised the role of families, included new language such as 'contracted service provider', and defined and clarified issues relating to the contracting out of services. This illustrated the emergence of the market in community care policy in Australia. There was a gradual shift towards a 'user pays' philosophy and an individualising of services. A Ministerial Task Force which reviewed intellectual disability services in 1995 recommended that 'the Government encourages strategies which allow clients, their families and the community to make some voluntary contribution towards services, should they wish to do so' (Intellectual Disability Services Task Force, 1995, p. 101). In practice, the voluntary nature of this recommendation in some instances was translated into families paying for additional services for their relatives who were in Government services. For example, one mother reported that she paid someone to take her son for a walk each week so that he could have some time away from the institution in which he lived. A housing study carried out by STAR, an advocacy group for people with intellectual disabilities and their families, found in 1995:

> an alarming trend by Health and Community Services towards a more aggressive application of the policy of families maintaining their relatives at home indefinitely. This policy was found to potentially be jeopardising the need and rights of adults under the Intellectually Disabled Persons' Services Act to achieve maximum independence. It also does not enable families, particularly parents, as they age, to be able to ever let go of their ongoing and often demanding caring and financial roles.

The Secretary of the Department responsible for intellectual disability services received publicity in 1992 for a statement in which he commented that 'advocacy is just pissing in the wind'. This view that advocacy was a luxury with little in the way of measurable outcomes was reflected in Government cuts to advocacy groups across the State. Only one advocacy organisation which was to represent all adult people with learning difficulties retained consistent government funding during this time. This had a number of effects: it robbed the Government and people with learning difficulties of a diversity of voices with which to argue different points of view. It split the advocacy movement into funded and unfunded groups. The Office of the Public Advocate received cuts to its services, reducing its capacity to undertake systemic advocacy. And the movement towards a focus on carers and the role of families gave parents a strong voice with Government, leading in some instances to a more conservative approach to people with learning difficulties.

The movement to close large institutions and to move people into the community continued, and two further large institutions in the state were closed. However the commitment to everyone with learning difficulties living in the community was mediated due to costs and changing ideologies. For example the closure of one large institution with approximately 500 residents led, for the first time in 20 years, to the building of a new institution for 104 residents on the site of the old institution. Described as a 'state of the art' residential service, the Government stated that it was to serve those people from the institution who 'chose' to live in an institutional setting or whose needs could not be met in the community. Both of these arguments were problematic in terms of rights.

New lives in a new century: 2000 and beyond

A new century saw a Labour Government in power in the state and a renewed interest in legislation relating to the needs of people with learning difficulties and in advocacy. The Intellectually Disabled Persons' Services Act has been reviewed and a new draft Disability Bill (Department of Human Services, 2006) is currently under discussion. The new Bill subsumes people with learning difficulties under the more general label of 'disability'. There are costs and benefits in this approach: it may reduce the negative labelling still attached to the term 'learning disabilities' and allow for a less restrictive approach to working with this group of people. However, it may also lead to a neglect of particular needs and interests experienced by people with learning difficulties. The new draft Act places a strong emphasis on increasing the involvement of people with disabilities in their communities. The first principle of the Act states that 'persons with a disability have the same basic rights and responsibilities as other members of the community and should be empowered to exercise these rights and responsibilities'.[5] A comparison with the corresponding principle in the Intellectually Disabled Persons' Services Act shows a continuing focus on rights but the introduction of the new term 'responsibilities' and a focus on empowerment of individuals rather than service delivery. The principles of the new draft Act place a greater emphasis on active participation and involvement by people with learning difficulties in their communities.

A new State Disability Plan 2002–12 was prepared and launched by the new Government after a more limited consultation than in the previous one. The vision expounded in the Plan is that:

> By 2012 Victoria will be a stronger and more inclusive community – a place where diversity is embraced and celebrated, and where everyone has the same opportunities to participate in the life of the community and the same responsibilities as all other citizens of Victoria. (Department of Human Services, 2002, p. 5)

The Plan sets as its goals the pursuit by people with disabilities of individual lifestyles, the building of 'inclusive communities' which are welcoming and accessible, the development of more inclusive and accessible public services and the promotion of non-discriminatory practices.

In practice the Government has developed a number of initiatives designed to put these goals into practice. For example programmes to strengthen and build participatory practices within government departments which are concerned with people with disabilities (Department of Human Services, 2005a), the development of disability action plans which are designed to increase opportunities for people with disabilities to gain employment, participate in consultation and decision making, improve staff awareness of their needs, provide accessible communication, information and services and improved physical access to buildings (Department of Human Services, 2005b), and policies designed to make the public transport system more accessible to people with disabilities (Department of Human Services, 2005c).

Deinstitutionalisation has continued with the current closure of the last of the large metropolitan institutions in the state. However, documentation of the closure process has shown that the focus on individual needs and interests demonstrated in the State Disability Plan and the Government initiatives has yet to be translated into practices of direct consultation with people with learning difficulties who were residents and the provision of community care designed to meet individual needs (Bigby, 2005).

It remains difficult to translate the ideals into practice on the ground. There has been a resurgence of interest in the role of advocacy for people with disabilities in the state. The Government has proposed the establishment of two units, a Disability Advocacy Unit and a Self Advocacy Resource Unit (Fyffe *et al.*, 2004a, b). These are designed to support and provide resources for advocacy and self advocacy organisations. At the time of writing, the development of these Units was being tendered out and their effectiveness in reinvigorating the advocacy organisations had yet to be tested.

Conclusion

Reflecting on the changes that have occurred in Victoria over the past 30 years has been a salutary exercise. What can be learnt from them? In terms of changing discourses, the language, policies and practices of Government and the community move swiftly and sometimes subtly. The language of rights which informed developments in the 1980s has been to some extent co-opted by a new discourse: deinstitutionalisation, community living, choice and family involvement are now terms used with a different emphasis and often a different meaning to that of the 1980s. The insertion of the term 'responsibilities' alone suggests a change in the way people with disabilities are now viewed by Government. As supporters of people with learning difficulties we need to be aware of these changes and be ready to either support or to offer a critique of their implications. We need to be able to use the current discourses in order to achieve support for people with learning difficulties to lead rewarding lives in the community.

With regard to changing community values and attitudes, the changes documented in this chapter reflect prevailing values and attitudes held more widely in the community. Outside of the field of learning difficulties, some writers in the USA, Britain and Australia have been documenting a movement towards increased individualism and a reduction in the focus on community values (Marquand, 1988; Lasch, 1995). The lessons from these writers and the critique of communities which they offer need to be taken seriously by people who work and advocate with people with learning difficulties. We need to consider seriously the kinds of communities in which people with learning difficulties are now living and to think about how theoretical analyses of the wider community can be used in developing policies and practices for them.

As for the importance of government, this chapter has revealed the importance of Government ideologies and practices in shaping the way people with learning difficulties are perceived and also how they may live their lives. Changes in Government have led to very different emphases on how services are provided in the community, in the degree of emphasis on participation and advocacy and in the movement of people with learning difficulties into the community.

Finally, in terms of rhetoric and action on the ground, in Victoria, there has been a shift to a more individualised focus to policy and planning and a concern about how to build inclusive communities. This is reflected in current Government policies and legislation. There are limits to how far these have had a direct impact on people's everyday lives. For example, Kirsten's narrative illustrates both the changes and the limits to them. Kirsten has lived through a time of rapid change in discourses affecting the lives of people with learning difficulties. From being designated a patient, someone who 'would never be any good', Kirsten came to be recognised as someone with a right to live in the community and to share in its life. However there were difficulties in this transition. There has been a continuing tendency to consider the needs of people with learning difficulties in terms of management of services, and although the focus on the individual and their needs and desires is becoming more apparent in some policy areas, in practice many people with learning difficulties continue to live in the community but not be a part of it. There is a need to now turn away from the idea of 'community care' with its suggestions of dependence and paternalism to one in which the life options of people with learning difficulties are taken seriously by those around them, and where there is an increasing focus on how to move communities to a more inclusive approach.

Change does not happen easily in the provision of services. It is even harder when it requires a fundamental shift in the way people are perceived and regarded by those around them. The position of many people with learning difficulties in Australian society has been changed. For such changes to be more than window dressing there still needs to be a lot of work done in changing views about them among the people who work closely with them and among other community members.

Notes

1. Kirsten was not able to tell her story directly. Rather the narrative was put together from 20 months' participant observation in the locked unit in the institution, interviews with staff and her mother, and reading the voluminous files which had been kept by the institution.
2. Intellectually Disabled Persons' Services Act, 1986.
3. Ibid.
4. Guardianship and Administration Board Act, 1986.
5. Disability Bill, Exposure Draft, p. 13.

Part IV

Experiences

In this part of the book, the perspectives of different stakeholders are examined. All the chapters draw on oral historical sources to illuminate how shifts to community care impacted upon, and were influenced by, individuals.

10
People with Learning Disabilities: Perspectives and Experiences

Katherine Owen and Sue Ledger

Introduction

This chapter presents three life stories. Through the stories we see how changing attitudes to care, control and citizenship have been experienced – how lives have been touched by the development of advocacy, patterns of migration, growth of market provision and changing models of support. These stories highlight the importance of sustained relationships, both from paid staff and more informal networks of friends, advocates and carers. We first describe the methodology used to construct the stories before presenting the stories themselves. The chapter concludes by exploring some of the central themes arising from the material presented and the methodology employed.

Methodology

The Introduction (pp. 1–14) has introduced the importance of life stories as a means of 'giving a voice' to people with learning disabilities, supplementing official history so that a further, more personal, dimension to historical issues is provided. Period detail is supplied through first-hand accounts. In this respect people with learning disabilities and their families are the experts (Sanderson, 2000). This presents fundamental challenges as to who has the right of ownership of a person's story and who determines the content. In this chapter, although using the term 'life story' to describe personal experience in general, we make the distinction between a life story which relies on the accounts of a primary narrator and a life history which combines different people's stories of an individual (Plummer, 1983, 1995; Goodley, 2000). The three life stories share the fundamental aim of wanting 'to understand people's direct understandings of the social worlds in which they live' (Plummer, 2001, p. 130) although they have been put together using different approaches.

The first, Anne's story, was originally presented as a pictorial autobiography, but individual photographs of sufficient quality for reproduction could not be extracted from the tape, and so this account focuses on the words extracted from the life story work. Initially Anne recorded memories of her life using a tape recorder. The tapes were transcribed and Anne identified gaps. The researchers then supported Anne to find archival material to fill in more of her story. Anne went back to visit the hospital where she had grown up, a former hostel and group home, and a video camera and photographs were used to record these visits. Using techniques adapted from reminiscence work (Schweitzer, 1993; Gibson, 1998) the photographs and video films were then watched with Anne which stimulated more memories. In this way Anne was supported to tell her own story. Anne herself retained control of the final version and was present at all visits to retrieve case records and archives.

The second story about Yvette is based on information recorded by Neil and Angela Harris, as part of the Witnesses to Change project (Rolph *et al.*, 2005). Neil and Angela knew Yvette as members of staff in the children's home where Yvette spent her childhood. They remained in contact, becoming close friends. Combining witness life histories in this way, creating a montage of memories to reconstruct missing pieces of history, has been successfully used by Rolph *et al.* (2005) when recording the experiences of families of people with learning disabilities. Such 'witness accounts' provided by family members, friends and advocates enable areas of shared experience and recurrent themes to be clearly identified.

Finally, Samantha's is a reconstructed life story. This is a method to tell the story of people who do not use words to communicate (Di Terlizzi, 1994). It uses data from field notes taken from participant observation with Samantha six months before and eighteen months after her move; interviews with her only remaining relative; interviews with members of staff both on the ward and in her new home; and analysis of documentation, including nurses' notes and assessments, from Samantha's past and present. In this way it follows a tradition of life stories gathered using ethnographic methods (Langness and Levine, 1986; Moore, 2004). It is a partial, or using Plummer's (2001) term, a 'topical' life story. It does not aim to capture the fullness of her life, but focuses on her move from institution into the community.

Anne's story

Anne's story was recorded in 2003–04. It speaks for itself – a powerful witness account of the changes in learning disability philosophy and services since 1948. The story documents the gradual change from a model of control delivered through long-stay hospital settings to a service-supported living model of service which endeavours to emphasise the individual's right to their own tenancy, everyday choices, and full involvement and control in planning their own future. Anne was born in 1948 and admitted to Normansfield Hospital in 1951 at the age of three, as a result of her epilepsy and 'associated difficult behaviours'. Anne's family sought a variety of highly respected medical opinions before taking this course of action. The family approached a Rudolf Steiner resource prior to Anne's admission to Normansfield, but Anne was not considered suitable due to the severity of her epilepsy.

Education at Normansfield was provided on site. There were few outings outside the hospital and Anne remembers spending a lot of time in the hospital ward undertaking a number of unpaid jobs caring for more highly dependent patients. Anne spent a total of 27 years in hospital. In 1977, Anne was offered the opportunity of resettlement to a room in a new local authority hostel located in the central London borough where her family lived. After several years in this large hostel, the offer of a room in a smaller, voluntary organisation, group home nearby followed. In 2004 Anne acquired the tenancy to her own flat. She is now involved with her local church and uses a wide variety of community resources such as colleges, library and local transport in addition to retaining involvement with groups used predominantly by people with learning disabilities such as People First and Gateway.

Yet, there are also continued sources of frustration for Anne. She has not been able to access paid employment in caring for animals or working with children as she would have wished and her income remains low. It is only recently that she has received any measure of success in trying to locate former friends from her years at Normansfield. After moving to the hostel, Anne participated in residents' meetings and later in advocacy meetings at the nearby SEC that she attended. This led on to active involvement in the local People First group and Anne remains a committed member. Anne has been involved in a number of local campaigns to improve services for people with learning disabilities.

The following words are extracted from Anne's life story work and accompanied the photographs in her life story book and the video images recorded on visits to the hospital where she had grown up, a local authority hostel, her previous group homes and a reunion with people she had known whilst a 'hospital patient':

Anne: This is my book and video. The pictures have helped me to remember the old days. I like to look at them. They make some people laugh and some people think it's sad what happened to me. The staff were very surprised when they saw it. They didn't know about the hospital. We took the photos of where I lived in the hospital I called the horrible old dump. The hospital was in Kingston outside London it wasn't easy for my family to visit. I have a map in my book – the hospital was here. I had to go to live at Normansfield when I was three years old. Because of my fits, I thought it was a horrible place. This is a picture of me when I was three when I went there. I was a little girl. This is a picture of the Stella Brain nursery at the hospital – I remember it there – we were all playing on the floor. I never went to proper school, only in the hospital. I lived on Spruce Ward. I remember that I had to help the nurses with the younger children. I also remember the theatre; we did some plays there and the theatre was also used for a church. The theatre is still there; I saw it when we went back. The hospital had big grounds and I used to go and hide from the nurses in the bushes. I left in 1977 – I remember visiting Piper House (a 25-bedded hostel in central London) and I thought this is better! My father was worried about my leaving hospital. He didn't want me to go. He thought I was safe there. But I said I'm going!

Gillian was my best friend in Normansfield. She came to visit me once after I left but she wasn't allowed to get out of hospital. I missed her. We lost touch. I would still like to find her. There was a residents group at the hostel and we talked about things. At Piper House I made some friends and we moved together to Colville Road (an 11 bedded voluntary sector group home). I liked it there but there was not enough space. My room was very small. In March this year I moved to my own flat but still live very near all my friends from the group home. I go to the local church and have a lot of friends there and at People First. I support Arsenal and go when I get the chance. I would still like a job with animals or working with little children.

Yvette's story

Yvette's story is based on transcripts of recordings with her two close friends. Neil and Angela Harris first met Yvette when they both worked as residential social workers in the 1970s and 1980s. Yvette grew up in the home where they worked and since she left they have remained in contact over many years. Yvette describes herself as a young, mixed-race woman with learning disabilities. She was born in central London in 1968. At birth she was diagnosed with Down's syndrome and so labelled as learning disabled from a very early age. She grew up in an inner London children's home in Chelsea.

Angela: I first got to know Yvette in 1979 when I went to work at the children's home, in Chelsea where Yvette was living. At that time there were 16 children there – can you believe? I was never her key worker or link worker – we had a link or key worker scheme at the time – I never had that sort of relationship with her. But I was always consistent because I was there until the point where she left and moved on to Crawley. During that time there were some staff who looked after her for the whole period but I was one of a group of people who consistently looked after her through her adolescence. They were important years – we met when Yvette was 11 and she left when she was 20.

Yvette was the only young person with a learning disability in the home. There was another young person who may have overlapped slightly with Yvette, she didn't have a learning disability but she was visually impaired. Yvette tended to socialise with the people from her school or the Gateway club. Yvette went to a Special School for young people with severe learning disabilities, Jack Tizard School. She wasn't in the mainstream education system. Some of the older children had their own rooms but on the whole the children had to share. I can remember Yvette shared with another young girl for a long time, probably four or five years. There were two of them in a bedroom. This girl did not have a learning disability and they were really good friends. This person came in after Yvette – they must have been about 13 years old when they started sharing. This young girl had two brothers who were also in the home and because she and Yvette were so close her brothers became very protective of Yvette too. Yvette saw these three very much as her close friends.

She was never bullied. She was always accepted. She was accepted for who she was, too. We didn't have any problems with accessing ordinary services such as the GP. Yvette has always been very able and keen to do things for herself. Yvette has always had a really strong character and was very much someone people knew locally. She would go out to the shops, as she got older; she might be in the local pub on a Friday night.

As Yvette had no family contact and no contact with anybody else outside the staff team and school, no independent bit at all, the local authority advertised specifically for a social aunt and uncle. But the idea of recruiting also came very much from Yvette because she felt that she didn't have anybody. The role of social aunt and uncle was almost like that of independent visitor today and perhaps a bit more as she used to go and stay overnight with these people. They were formally assessed and approved as social aunt and uncle before being introduced to Yvette. The people selected were a white Irish family. The fostering team organised this. She would see them about once a month. They would come and visit her at the home and go out with her and if there was any special event going on in the family she would often join in.

Yvette then moved to Crawley. It was thought best for her to live out of the city. But it entailed many losses of the contacts which had sustained her through her childhood.

Angela: It was funny because there was this consistent core of people who had cared for her throughout her adolescence and there was also, very importantly, the support staff. The cleaners – there were three of them and they all knew Yvette very well and were very fond of her.

Neil: Because she had been at the home so long Yvette really was part and parcel of the nuts and bolts of the place and I can remember it was myself who drove Yvette to Crawley with her link worker at the time. The day she left it was awful, everyone was in tears. The cleaners were in tears and the staff. There was this whole line up of people saying goodbye and crying. And I was trying to make it something positive about Yvette starting her new life ...

If we think about it, the potential for not-so-good outcomes for Yvette is immense. She's been rejected by some very important key people in her life who have left her. And she moved out of what had been her environment, her networks and locality, to Crawley. She could have been very unhappy and isolated but she's not and that's down to her force of character.

I wasn't involved in the decision making at the time but I know there was a big debate about risk and risk management, particularly in the context of living in inner London as it was seen. But Yvette had all her links there and although things have all turned out very well in Crawley now and Yvette is very happy and has been very successful, I think in retrospect it probably was the wrong decision. I know there was a debate. On the one hand, Yvette has the children's home, where she had lived for many years, as a base to come back to, and she had all her connections with the Gateway club and other organisations in the area, mainly for people with learning disabilities where she was very involved. On the other hand there was concern about her travelling alone and 'London being a dangerous place'. Sadly I think in many ways the fact that Yvette had some independence worked against her. I think it very much was the practice of the time for the best reasons people somehow thought people like Yvette would be 'better in the country'. At that point she didn't have any one who was clearly her advocate, someone who was there solely for her. I think that all the people around her for all the right reasons perhaps made the wrong decision. Yes, if she had been consulted properly and her views taken seriously into account she wouldn't have gone.

The move was extremely traumatic for Yvette and it took her a long, long time and many, many years to settle into Crawley and every time we saw her in the early days she would say how she didn't like it. And then she would come up to us for the weekend and she'd want to phone the children's home. She'd want to find out all the news from the manager.

Angela: I was quite friendly with Yvette's link worker at the time of her move to Crawley so when she would be going down to visit Yvette in her new home I'd go along. This was only occasionally, it might be only every six months, say. But then the turning point of it was when she became very ill and her Crohn's Disease was diagnosed. She was in hospital for a lot of weeks, perhaps about six weeks. She was really ill and lost a tremendous amount of weight.

Continued

She was in an isolation ward for a while. She really was extremely ill. So during that time I went down to see her more often. At that time she really didn't have anybody of her own and that was the first point really when I said to her 'why don't you come up for a weekend?' And that was where it started really. Yvette began visiting us at our home for the day and then for overnight stays.

Yvette still lives in Crawley where she now has her own flat, circle of friends and a job she enjoys.

Neil and Angela: I think now Yvette's life is transformed. She has a job and hopefully she will soon get paid for it. She has her own flat, which is something that she has always wanted. This was her ambition even as a teenager. I think the flat was a real turning point for Yvette settling in Crawley – after she got her own flat it became her real home. She's got her friends now a widening circle. It's taken time but she got there. There are people like us, and her social aunt and uncle whom she still keeps in touch with, sees regularly and regards as family. We see Yvette as a very close friend of our family; we will always stay in touch. Its difficult, as I think there was a period in her life from the age of 20 for about ten years or so, when I don't think she was happy.

Yvette has not had contact with her natural family since she was a child. Neil and Angela reflect on her life and the decisions made about it. They comment on how the care planning system of the time weighed concerns about risk against factors such as social links, ethnicity and culture when it was decided that Yvette should leave London.

Neil and Angela: At the children's home there would be a meeting about twice a year. When I think of the records that were kept then, it was so different. There wasn't a care plan. It was well before the Children Act. I think her social worker was very happy for Yvette to stay at the children's home as she was happy there. Although she was happy no one seemed to be thinking what's it going to be like in ten, fifteen years time. The planning seemed to go instead from meeting to meeting. Long-term fostering seemed to take a long time to arrange then and was not pursued across the board as actively as it is now. Whereas if long-term fostering had been pushed for many of the children, including Yvette, it may have given them wider social networks later on. Or even if she had have stayed in Chelsea, moving to local accommodation, I think she would have developed a wider network of people more quickly as she had existing contacts to build on, whereas in Crawley

Continued

she had to start from scratch. Although saying that now, after all these years, Yvette is beginning to catch up in this respect and she has a wider circle of people …

Neil: If I could have changed things in terms of how things were arranged for Yvette, and from our ongoing friendship with Yvette throughout the years, I would have liked her to be given more credit. I think an independent advocate would have been really helpful for Yvette when she was younger and having to make decisions about where she would move to after the children's home. Nowadays I don't feel Yvette would need an advocate, just someone to sit down and listen carefully to what she thinks and says and take that very seriously.

I think that the care given to Yvette was consistent and protective but it was almost an attitude of 'we know what's best, what's good for you'. I think that if more work had been done with Yvette on her cultural background then it might have helped her develop more of a sense of 'who I am, where I'm from and where I might be going'. Issues of people's ethnic and cultural backgrounds were not really spoken about then – not with the young people themselves. God knows why, but people didn't think to do things like life story books with kids then. Yvette would have been a wonderful person to do something like that with. As carers in a children's home we had very little information about Yvette's background … .

Neil and Angela: *When I first met Yvette there was some letter contact with her family but then that stopped and there was none at all. In all the time we worked alongside Yvette we don't remember any discussion of her cultural heritage. Yvette's natural mother is white and her father Caribbean. I can't remember any specific piece of work or focus on that. This was I think unfortunately quite common then. The focus was more on the issue of difficulty*

In Crawley, Yvette moved from a registered care home to her own tenancy and from day care provided by the local authority in a SEC to a voluntary sector organisation and subsequently to work experience. She has her own flat, a support package which she is actively involved in directing and has begun setting up a Direct Payment. She has a job at a local supermarket and attends mainstream further education evening classes, a local gym, and keep fit classes. Yvette exercises her right to vote. Yvette's health care needs and screening are all met through local primary and acute services. In this way we can see some of the influence of changing policy direction, such as the Direct Payments Act, 1996 (DOH, 2001a), and how it affects the way support is delivered. Yvette is still aiming to obtain full-time employment converting her work experience job to fully paid work. Neil and Angela have the last word:

We feel very, very proud of Yvette. When she comes to stay we will generally always meet up with our extended family. We will meet up for a dinner or maybe go out and she is so relaxed, respectful and nice to people. By the way she behaves and acts it shows she has been really well brought up. In the end it's all worked out very well.

Samantha's story

Although moving people with learning difficulties out of long-term institutional care has been Government policy for the best part of 50 years, in 2001 some 1500 people still lived in long-stay hospitals (DOH, 2001a). By definition, these people were seen as the most difficult to place in the community, perhaps due to having more severe learning difficulties, complex needs, mental health problems and/or challenging behaviour. This life history is the story of one such woman, Samantha Hill, who moved into a community home in 2000. She was described as having severe learning difficulties and challenging behaviour and had lived in long-term institutional care since the age of five. Her story offers an opportunity to make a comparison between her life before and after her move into the community.

When I (Katherine Owen) first met Samantha she was 52 years old and had lived on Greenfield ward, a locked ward in a hospital, for over ten years. I met her while conducting fieldwork for a three-year ethnographic study which aimed to understand the experience of women with severe learning difficulties moving out of a locked ward into community homes (Owen, 2004). She was one of eleven women in the study whom I spent time with as they moved out of Greenfield Ward. I have chosen to highlight her story for several reasons. First, only three of the women in the study moved to residential care homes in the community. The others were considered 'too dangerous' and therefore remained in an NHS campus home in the grounds of the hospital. Second, of those three women, Samantha's story outlines a more 'ordinary' experience. Her move led neither to a dramatic change for the better in her life, nor to a change for the worse. Finally, her story highlights how often change for the better for people moving to the community is incremental, fragile and heavily dependent on the skills, values and attitudes of the staff who support them.

Her life story is reconstructed, using data from a variety of different sources (Di Terlizzi, 1994). These include fieldnotes written during participant observation with Samantha conducted 6 months before and 18 months after her move into a community home, interviews with her aunt (her only remaining relative), and with members of staff both on the ward and in her new home, and finally an analysis of documentation, including nurses' notes and assessments, from her past and present.

Samantha was born in London in 1947. She was a beautiful little girl, said by her aunt to be, 'like a doll', with curly blond hair and clear, pale skin. Her parents were described as having 'real affection for their child' (written by a doctor in 1952). Her father, in particular, 'adored her' and 'idolised her'. Her aunt described how when Samantha was a baby her father used to massage her in olive oil on the kitchen table. However, Samantha was slow to develop and started to have 'fits'. When she was five she was admitted for long-term care because her parents were unable to cope with her 'restless and destructive behaviour'. In 1951, she was described as being:

> an untamed animal, wandering about, interfering with the pupils and nothing is safe within her grasp. She tears up papers, etc., and hits other children ... If restrained in any way she resorts to fits of screaming and temper, pulling at her hair and hitting herself. She is dirty in her habits.[1]

Samantha's parents continued to take an active part in her life, visiting her weekly, until their deaths in the mid-1980s and early 1990s. Samantha lived in at least three different hospitals. She had spent 36 years in the hospital in which she lived now, although during this time she had moved between numerous wards.

Samantha was a small, almost delicate, woman, who liked to keep herself to herself, and was almost constantly on the go. She did not use speech to communicate apart from saying 'yes' and 'no' occasionally. She was one of the most vulnerable women on the ward and was often covered in cuts and bruises caused by the other women. Samantha was on a locked ward due to her foraging for food and cigarette ends, and other 'challenging behaviour'. Her life was one of routine and structure, with set times for getting up, having baths, eating meals and getting cups of tea. She spent the majority of her time waiting by the kitchen door just in case there was a moment when a staff member would make her an 'extra' cup of tea, or by the locked front door, waiting for an opportunity to be able to get outside.

She enjoyed going out, and sometimes went for walks around the hospital grounds. She also had 1:1 sessions at the specialist day service for people with autism, which lasted for 20 minutes twice a week. At these times she was encouraged to do art and craft, or relax in the Snoezelen room. The rest of the time she spent on the ward. Most rooms were locked (including her bedroom), although the two main communal areas, the living room and dining room, were always open. However, Samantha wanted time and space alone, which meant she frequently stood in the corridors. She often seemed on edge, would pace up and down, and breathe quickly and noisily, often waiting for a moment when she would have to move quickly to get something that she wanted. On the ward, Samantha was seen by the staff to be a 'good girl' because she was not loud or violent with others. She was considered to be 'naughty' if she disobeyed the rules, for example getting up from her seat during mealtimes, or taking food or drink from other people. She was very focused on getting her needs met and was respected by the majority of the staff for her determination.

Samantha moved to a large residential care home, Plum House, in the summer of 2000. From the start there was more flexibility in her daily routine in the new home. She could have cups of tea throughout the day, go to bed when she was tired and have snacks if she made it known she was hungry. However, she continued to have no say in when she got up in the morning. She was dependent on the shift patterns of the staff and would wait for them each morning crouched down behind her bedroom door. There was also the possibility for Samantha to be more involved in some of her daily routines. In her new home Samantha was supported to wash and dress each morning by a single member of staff. This meant that the staff member had more time to find out how she was and what her wishes were on any given day. Samantha was able to choose whether she stood up or sat down to be washed. When she returned to her bedroom, there was opportunity for her to be part of the process of getting dressed.

She no longer went to a day service, but had her daytime activities planned by the staff in her home. However, she had a limited choice and the activities she got involved in did not really suit her interests. What she did seemed to depend on the activities of other residents, so she went on trips on the bus when others needed collecting or was taken trampolining which she did not enjoy. There was little opportunity for her to discover new experiences or learn new skills, let alone engage with others. She did, however, get out more. She enjoyed walks up to the local high street for a cup of tea. She began to be known by the waitress in a café who would make her a cup of tea, just the way she liked it. Samantha would also go to the supermarket where she would get extra milk for the house or other items that were needed.

She experienced more freedom in other areas of her life too. Although the front door was locked at all times, she could go up to her bedroom at any time in the day (although this was not encouraged as it was at these times that she sometimes became destructive). The kitchen door was also locked and she used to wait outside it as she had done on Greenfield ward. The staff realised her need for tea, but also acknowledged that it would not be good for her to have it as often as she wanted, so tried her with decaffeinated options.

There was evidence to suggest she was listened to more. She was seen as an individual with rights and needs. If she took food from another person's plate, the staff concluded that she was hungry and got her some more food. If it was hot and she began to take her clothes off, she would be offered a cool shower, a cold drink or some lighter clothes. Instead of being forced to have her hair cut to fit into the timings or requirements of others, she was treated with patience and respect. If necessary it was decided to 'try again another time', to wait until she 'was ready'. Thus she was not punished for being 'naughty' or made to go without to teach her a lesson.

Some things changed little. Samantha had limited choice over what she ate. Mealtimes in Plum House were very similar to Greenfield ward. They were mainly functional with little emphasis on enjoyment or spending time together. Staff and residents would eat separately, and residents finished their food as quickly as possible. Staff only sat with the residents during mealtimes for practical purposes (to help someone eat) and on those occasions their chairs would be placed at right angles to the table. However, for Samantha, there was more opportunity to choose where she sat each day and to be given something different to eat if she did not like what had been served.

Samantha had no choice of whom she lived with. She lived with more people than she did before and with men as well as women. She still experienced violence. On one visit, she came to sit beside me and burst into tears. I was told that a resident had kicked her and that was why she was crying. Relationships between residents were encouraged by staff. They would organise for the other residents to give Samantha a birthday card. She seemed to spend more time with others in communal rooms. She often seemed more relaxed, and would sit beside people on the sofa and doze. In terms of relationships with people outside the house, her social networks remained narrow and her potential to be lonely remained.

Finally, Samantha was more consistently acknowledged as an adult woman. This was reflected in her appearance, for example, her selection of new clothes, which were smart and appropriate for a woman in middle age. She loved to have her make up done. Staff described how she would turn her head towards them in order to make it easier to apply; she would also hold still, even long enough for her nails to be painted. It was also the first time she consistently wore a bra.

Summary

Samantha's life in her new home changed for the better in many ways. It demonstrates how positive change for people with severe learning disabilities is often dependant on the staff around them. Staff who value the rights of people with learning difficulties and who see people as individuals with their own wishes, desires and emotional life are essential. But Samantha's new life was a long way from the 'full and rewarding' life promised in *Valuing People*. Samantha's life in the community, although improved, did not match the vision of a modern society in which 'everyone is valued and has the chance to play their full part' (DOH, 2001a).

Conclusion

These three life stories highlight the struggle that people with learning disabilities have encountered in getting their voices heard and their wishes respected. In terms of housing, care, advocacy and policy they demonstrate a gradual shift to improved community provision. However, they also highlight how, several years after *Valuing People*, and an explicit commitment by the Government to implement the Disability Discrimination Act (1995, 2005) and Human Rights (1998) legislation, some people with learning disabilities continue to struggle with exclusion and discrimination which prevent them from experiencing citizenship in its fullest sense.

In current services, life story work is receiving increasing recognition in approaches to service delivery which emphasise citizenship and the need to hand back control to the individual (Sanderson, 1998, 2000; Sanderson *et al.*, 2002). Although time consuming, this trend represents a shift away from case records (Gillman *et al.*, 1997) and the medicalisation of learning disability, to an approach based on the social model of disability. The telling/writing of the life story can have an impact at both a personal and social level. At a personal level, it presents the ideal opportunity for people to look back and make sense of their own lives. The act of story telling involves them in the all-important process of life review. This can be an empowering process. For people who do not use speech the process of review is equally important, enabling valuable life story information to be recorded and shared with significant others.

At a social level, life stories can highlight commonalities as well as differences. This includes experiences which are shared with other people with learning difficulties as well as with the rest of society. Bersani (1998) has suggested that this sharing of experience has the potential to encourage people with learning disabilities to develop a social awareness and understanding of the sources and meaning of those shared experiences and so begin to see themselves as part of a 'social movement'. It also has the potential to involve the rest of us in developing a greater understanding of people's lives and to be enriched by that understanding.

Note

1. The referral report to the long-stay hospital.

11
The Role and Perspectives of Families

Sheena Rolph

Introduction

Although it is recognised that families have always been central to the care of people with learning difficulties, their role and agency in the second half of the twentieth century in challenging policies and promoting change has only recently begun to be explored. When historians in the 1990s began to look outside institutional history, they found evidence, not only of links between institutions and community, but of active families engaging with national and local policies, sometimes colluding with, sometimes challenging them (Digby and Wright, 1996; Thomson, 1996, 1998a; Melling *et al.*, 1997; Wright, 1998; Bartlett and Wright, 1999). More recently, the role and influence of families in twentieth-century community care is being further evaluated in countries such as Canada (Christie and Gauvreau, 2004; Chupik and Wright, 2006); Australia, New Zealand and several European countries (Traustadottir and Johnson, 2000); and Britain (Walmsley and Rolph, 2001; Rolph, 2002, 2005a–f; Rolph *et al.*, 2005). In the main, these authors highlight the continuity of the role of the family in providing care in the community.

This chapter explores this continuing centrality of the family in the lives of people with learning difficulties (Traustadottir and Johnson, 2000; Walmsley and Rolph, 2001), and its place within the changing and developing concepts of control, care and citizenship. In particular, it focuses on what happened when parents assumed a new role after the Second World War, banding together for the first time in local Mencap Societies with the aim of challenging segregative and discriminatory government policies. Although policy changes were slow to arrive, families responded by setting up new services themselves, side-stepping local authority control on the one hand, and prevarication and neglect on the other. On occasion, alliances between families and local government officers were able to impact upon local policies, as were campaigns, lobbying and activism. This chapter also asks whether changes of policy, combined with the new rights and citizenship agenda, made any real improvement in the lives of people with learning difficulties and their families. It uses the oral history testimonies of families themselves to interrogate these issues, foregrounding their stories.

Issues in the research methodology

The chapter draws on the author's extensive work in carrying out oral history interviews with families and people with learning difficulties. The aim is to contribute a rounded picture which will include not only the achievements of families, but also the difficulties which confronted them. Responses vary from the testimonies of the Mencap activists, to the day-to-day stories of families who were not involved politically with movements of any kind, to those of families who, for many different reasons, struggled to care effectively for their children. The challenge for oral history researchers in the field of learning disability is to tell all three parallel stories (Rolph and Walmsley, 2006). The dilemma is that we hear a great deal from families in the first two groups who, given the opportunity, are eager to tell their stories which are often accounts of hardship and lack of provision on the one hand, but also of progress and milestones on the other. We are less likely to hear from those parents at the end of their tether who, for a variety of reasons, including despair, poverty, ignorance or shame and the lack of any meaningful support, neglected to care effectively for their children (French, 1972).

Significantly, now that people with learning difficulties themselves are beginning to talk and write about their lives, stories of mistreatment or neglect by families are beginning to emerge (Atkinson and Williams, 1990). Cissy Negus has described her home situation in Cambridge during the War:

> We had a cruel Mum. She used to shut us up with a stick. She used to shut us up in the bedroom, me and Sonny and Lily and Rene and Daisy. We all got shut in the bedroom. She wouldn't let us come down, either. (Rolph, 2005a, p. 64)

For the children involved, these were terrible situations. For young parents, alone and stigmatised, often without any help from the visiting officers under the Mental Deficiency Acts who were sometimes more judgemental than supportive (Walmsley, 1994; Rolph, 2000) tensions often became unbearable (Hall and Rolph, 2005). In a chapter devoted to the central role of families in community care, it is important to be aware of the possibility of stereotypes, idealisation and myths and to acknowledge that there have also always been families who were sometimes not able to carry out this caring role, to the detriment of their children. Although dominant narratives have emerged in the history of learning disability, there are also these individual testimonies which are emerging to challenge them and which help to build a more complete picture. These demurring narratives – in this case those of children or siblings – are not often told, or incorporated alongside the dominant testimonies, to modify and explore them (Green, 2004).

A new role for families 1946–59: the emergence of local voluntary Societies

This section explores the role played by some of those families who were more active and politically engaged, with an account of the development of local voluntary Societies and their contribution to community care in the second half of the twentieth century. Due to the fact that the primary research for this chapter has been based in England, these are the stories of Mencap activists, but there is no reason to believe they do not represent the experiences of people in other countries of the UK and beyond (Trent, 1994). The section is based largely on oral history work carried out in East Anglia with seven local Mencap Societies (Rolph, 2002, 2005a–f). Geographically the research is therefore well grounded in a local context, which enables a detailed focus on the activities of local families associated with the Societies. Although it is not possible to generalise from local studies to a national picture, it is likely that studies in East Anglia may well reflect some of the developments in other areas of the UK.

Studies of the interwar period have highlighted the paradoxical position of the family within the mental deficiency legislation: on the one hand it was the stigmatised source of perceived hereditary problems (Tredgold, 1908; Macnicol, 1987); on the other it was to play an important role in the community care provisions of the Acts (Thomson, 1998a). Families were visited by officials who had to balance the duties of care and control and who were often greeted with suspicion by families (Walmsley and Rolph, 2001, pp. 71–2). Although on the face of it families did not have much control over their lives in this period, Thomson has pointed out ways in which they were on occasion able to get the better of the authorities and sometimes even colluded with them (Thomson, 1996).

Nevertheless, there was little provision for their children in the community, a situation parents aimed to rectify after the War. The year 1946 saw the start of a new grassroots voluntary movement in England which began to work and campaign in the community to regain some power over their own lives and those of their children and, in the light of the huge gaps in community provision, to provide their own forms of benign community care. The National Association of Parents of Backward Children (NAPBC) founded in 1946, and later known as Mencap, is well known. As well as the national society, however, hundreds of local Mencap Societies were also set up in the following years, taking issue with mainly controlling local and national policies (Rolph, 2002, 2005a–f). They provided the forum for a new role for parents and an opportunity for them to try to influence policy (Walmsley, 2000a). The extent to which voluntary organisations were successful in this aim is debatable. However, there is no doubt that this was their intention, and many of the families interviewed for the research believed their campaigning had changed policies and attitudes significantly, either at the local or national level.

As in the USA (Trent, 1994), various factors coming together in the immediate postwar period acted as powerful catalysts prompting families at last to group together to fight for justice and equality for their sons and daughters and to create and lobby for community services to replace institutional care – for some, though not all, a major consideration (Rolph *et al.*, 2005). The often painful and difficult role undertaken by families has been underestimated, and one aspect in particular of their emerging ideas and ideology has gone unnoticed in the literature. Testimonies indicate that many families influential in local Societies anticipated the social model of disability by some decades in their identification of society – not their learning disabled children – as the problem. In the second half of the century, families aimed to make an impact on the local communities they lived in, either informally (through becoming more visible) or more formally through Year Books and cine films (Rolph, 2005e). In these photographs and films, their children were not depicted in institutions or as medical cases as so often before (Tredgold, 1908; Shuttleworth and Potts, 1910; Herd, 1930) but were seen in ordinary situations, at parties, on outings or at work – and for the time this was breaking serious taboos. These early (1950s) public displays of photographs and films were a way of asserting the ordinariness of their children, set against society's prejudices. Brenda Nickson identified society as the problem for her son, stating as the aim of the new Society:

> To try and get support and recognition ... and to try and get people to treat our children as though there was at least a certain amount of

normality in all – they were all human beings. To try and get them recognised as people ... so that they were not different to the extent that they were originally looked on as being different ... I think that was the biggest aim the Society was trying to achieve. (Rolph, 2005b, p. 30)

'Pushing an empty pram': testimonies and silences

Oral history testimonies reveal some of the issues that faced individual families after the War. According to Brenda Nickson:

> When our son was born, I was just told that he was a 'Mongol', as they were called in those days, and there would be no future for him, and he'd probably not live longer than five. They said the best thing for us to do was to put him in an institution. Needless to say my husband and I were so horrified we just picked up our bags and left. I had a good weep, of course. I think I spent the first two years crying. We were just left then. At that time nobody acknowledged you. (Nickson, 2005, p. 77)

This obfuscation and the delays in diagnosis were compounded by public attitudes which added to feelings of isolation. Although it was the task of DAOs, and their successors MWOs, to visit families as regularly as possible, the visits were infrequent owing to the huge workloads of the officers, who in any case could offer little in the way of support other than a place in an institution (Rolph *et al.*, 2003). Vi Hardy's family had only one disappointingly brief encounter with an MWO:

> A Mental Welfare Officer visited to help Margaret [Vi's daughter] who at the time was crawling about on the floor. She gave Margaret a toy to help her use her fingers. Vi said: 'What a marvellous idea'. It was little pegs to go into holes. The visitor said 'I will call to see Margaret in a fortnight'. Vi next saw her in eleven months' time. She was really useless. (Hardy, 2005, pp. 41–2)

Lilian Fisher, on the other hand, described the excitement and apprehension she felt before the first meeting of the Lowestoft Mencap Society in 1962:

> I walked into the room and felt quite nervous. Who would be there? Who would I meet? Yet I felt this was the way forward. There was a coming together of parents with a handicapped child with the aim of

helping ourselves and each other. How wonderful it was to meet them and to know we were not alone. (Fisher, 2005, pp. 91–2)

Associated with the need to change attitudes was the strength of feeling about the *rights* of their children which was in evidence at a very early stage, as recalled by several founder members of the Societies. Societies took on the task of enabling change in different ways, sometimes by simply appearing in public on holidays and outings, sometimes by sharing holiday venues for the first time with the general public. Often, they encountered discrimination and sometimes abuse from the public. But gradually, they began to achieve some success, as remembered on one occasion by the founder member of a Society:

> We went to a holiday camp on the Isle of Wight. And of course there was the general public there as well. We took about a dozen or so of us and we heard this remark from a family: 'I wish we hadn't come this week, there are some handicapped people up there'. But at the end of the week, the family turned round ... and bought us a bottle of champagne! ... That was one of the best holidays. (Martin Brown quoted in Rolph, 2005c, p. 46)

Society holidays therefore had a hidden agenda: as well as being great fun, they also became experiments in integration.

Sometimes there were family silences after the birth of a baby, as some members of the family suspected that something was wrong but did not voice their fears. Sometimes the initial silences within families were then echoed by the need to hide from the outside world. Reaction from other mothers or people in the street was often ambiguous and hurtful. Another mother said: 'And when you went out with the baby, you just felt you were pushing an empty pram because people didn't know what to say to you' (Nickson, 2005, p. 77). One mother remembered that the Headmistress at the local Infant School asked if she would like to send her son to the school: 'I said "Yes, of course" and he was there for a little while, but then some of the parents said they didn't think he should be there. It was very difficult to say the least. I must admit ... we felt very lonely' (Abbs, 2005, p. 38). Such attempts to render children with learning difficulties invisible were exacerbated by an education policy experienced by many parents as segregating and excluding.

'Classified as ineducable': education policy

Parents were frustrated by a postwar education policy which still excluded many of their children from both ordinary and Special

Schools, judging them to be 'ineducable'. Children assessed as having an IQ of 50 or above could attend Special Schools, while those with an assessment below this were described by the Act as 'ineducable' and could only attend an Occupation Centre. Many parents experienced this discriminatory practice. Exclusion from Special School was one of the most painful experiences of parents and was felt to be unjust and discriminatory. Bedford LEA wrote to Brenda Nickson in September 1959, spelling out both a judgement on her son and the types of alternative provision on offer:

> I ... write to give you the formal notice that the Authority have come to the conclusion that your son is suffering from a disability of the mind of such a nature and to such an extent as to make him incapable of receiving education at an ordinary or special school. It is the duty of the Local Health Authority to do all they can to help a child concerning whom such a report is issued. Such help may take the form of visits by and advice from Mental Health Workers, provision of instruction at home at the Centres, or arrangements for the provision of residential accommodation.[1]

Betty Colby, who worked at the Great Yarmouth Occupation Centre after the War, remembered her other role as community visitor:

> We used to go round visiting the handicapped children that couldn't go to school, just to see that they were looked after. Some of the families were in poor straits, some of them were very poor things. But we couldn't offer an awful lot of help in those days. Sometimes on a Saturday morning I was called in to go and visit somebody. Perhaps a mother would be a bit worried about a child and we would just go round. But there was nothing much that you could do really, just talk to them. (Rolph, 2005c)

Until 1962 there were no Special Schools or special classes in Lowestoft, Suffolk. Instead, the local authority relied on open air classes at three ordinary schools, and the Occupation Centre (Wilmot and Saul, 1998; Lowe, 2003). Neville Porter, as a newly appointed MWO, described his first visit to the Occupation Centre (later JTC), working with the newly formed Lowestoft Society to improve provision:

> When I first went to Lowestoft [in the early 1950s], we had the most atrocious training centre for children until they were 16 or 17. It was an old church hall where the roof leaked. It was so bad that, after lots of pushing, we opened a small centre at Warren Road.[2]

This Training Centre was also only for the more physically able children which left many parents in despair at the lack of help. Families lived in dread of the designation of 'ineducable' being used by the authorities to place the children under supervision in their homes or to enter their child into an institution. Education for their children remained patchy and sparse, especially in rural counties, and families depended on the weekly visits of the home teacher and on daily or sometimes only fort-nightly Occupation Centres. Other local Societies began to open their own Occupation Centres and Training Centres, as well as crèches for younger children, and they campaigned for improvements in local authority-run centres and JTCs. In the face of the injustices with regard to education – and the appalling condition of some of the few Occupation Centres – Societies began to engage with local authority departments, spurred on by their belief in the abilities, educability, and rights of their children. Even so, families had to wait many years before the education of their children was considered a right, and before this was recognised in government policy, as discussed in Chapter 4.

'People's lives depended on it'

There were other less tangible achievements in the early years of the Societies. As one Lowestoft member said, 'the Societies opened windows and doors' for the members (Rolph, 2002). One of the most important functions of the Societies was to raise morale and give confidence to families. Friendship, acceptance and moral support were the vital in-gredients. Societies set up welfare visiting schemes with the aim of supporting all families, whether members of Mencap or not. For many families, the Societies provided the means to have a new life and to feel useful and needed by their local communities. Organisational and fund-raising skills and many other talents became indispensable. Fund-raising events were crucial to the continued existence and success of the Societies, and, as one mother said:

> we could use all sorts of talents that had lain dormant for years ... Suddenly we realised we weren't on our own ... it was a great relief, we thought we must be the only parents struggling like that ... The society helped to get rid of embarrassment and stigma because it was talked about, it was in the open ... You weren't at home brooding over the sit-uation, wondering what was going to happen – we made things hap-pen. It was always lively – and people's lives depended on it. It gave us all a purpose. (Fisher in Rolph, 2002, p. 45)

Perceptions of families over this time changed: from the guilty perpetrators of social ills to people who were to be pitied, from a 'social problem group' to 'problem families' in the 1950s (Macnicol, 1987; Welshman, 1996, 1999b); and from 'a nuisance group' to 'a force to be reckoned with'. They gradually began to be perceived as people 'burdened with care', deserving of sympathy and support. Partly this was due to the discrediting of eugenic ideas during the Second World War; partly to media attention and autobiographies by parents emphasising their plight and asking for sympathy (Hannam, 1975; McCormack, 1978; Boston, 1981; Hebden, 1985). The Societies were 'both the symbol and cause of shifting perceptions' (Walmsley, 2001). They used the 'pitiable' Little Stephen logo on their publicity and Year Books to raise money, and to gain sympathy rather than abuse, insisting that their children were people first, deserving of an ordinary life and equality of opportunity and services. At this stage, however, the publicity of the National Society aimed to evoke pity rather than respect and care rather than citizenship. Significantly, during the lead-up to the 1959 Mental Health Act, the local Societies began to be included in policy debates at national level. The NAPBC was asked to participate in discussions leading to the Act, and to make proposals to the 1954–57 Royal Commission set up to debate the issues. In the event, the Act promised much but delivered little, and several more decades of campaigning and lobbying still lay ahead of families and Societies.

'We didn't depend on anybody': parents as carers and advocates: 1959–71

Although this was a period of transition, of a policy switch to increasing care in the community, of changing labels, families still found that they had much to struggle for, and voices of resistance were dominant. The situation remained unsatisfactory for many families, and Mencap Societies retained their pivotal position in both providing services and lobbying for more. Although the long-stay hospitals continued to grow in size during this period until 1969, their eventual closure began to be seen as inevitable. This meant that families were once again identified as the main carers, given that services to replace the hospitals were not yet in place. They were often left to cope with little support (Bayley, 1973; McCormack, 1978; Wilkin, 1979; Rolph, 2002, 2005a–f; Rolph *et al.*, 2005). Some typical comments from the period are: '... we had a hard time of it. We never expected anybody to do things for us, we did it for ourselves ... We didn't depend on anybody. We never had social workers' (Winder in Rolph *et al.*, 2005, p. 186). One mother did have visits from a health worker which she describes as being very unsatisfactory:

> She was useless. She used to come and have a cup of tea or coffee. She wasn't interested in Christine's welfare at all. Never discussed it – just wanted to talk about general things. So she was hopeless. That's the only thing I got from the welfare. And I remember one time, something was announced that they were going to give people help. They came along and asked me would I like two pounds of sugar and a pound of butter! They offered me that! I threw them out. That was the help I've had from the welfare. (Rolph, 2005c, p. 37)

Parents increasingly assumed the role of advocates for their children (Rolph *et al.*, 2005, p. 216). Josey Griffin summed up what she saw as the pioneering work of the Society in the years before 1970:

> I think the important thing was that it did actually persuade the local authorities to start doing things that were needed. Up to then it was something that they virtually turned a blind eye to. And I think as it developed, they started getting a guilty conscience. It didn't happen for a long time, but it just triggered things off. It made them recognize the sort of things that were necessary. (Rolph, 2005b, pp. 58–9)

Moves towards inclusive education

Significantly, in the 1960s some interesting experiments in integrated education were promoted by parents. Families initiated the idea of Opportunity Classes – usually nursery classes for those children with severe learning difficulties – which began to be set up in different parts of the country. One example was a class which opened in Stevenage in 1966 (Payne, 1969). It was a twice-weekly Class and, crucially, the children were joined by the pre-school children of the volunteer staff, together with other children from the local nursery school, creating an integrated class. The aim was 'to enable handicapped children to mix with children who are free from handicap' (Faulkner, 1969). Dr Ron Faulkner noted that:

> the children benefit from ... the socialising pressure of membership of a group of children ... some of our children go on from the Opportunity Class to attend morning sessions of our sponsoring Nursery School ... There is no doubt that some of our former

members who are now attending, for example an ESN School would, without the Opportunity Class, have been assessed at a lower level. (Faulkner, 1969)

Interestingly, this class also enabled parents to have some experience in the actual planning of services. Educational experiments such as that at Roehampton pre-empted further significant developments in the final period under review.

Debates concerning rights and citizenship: 1970–2001

In the period 1970–2001, culminating in *Valuing People*, the family's role in community care has been further emphasised in policy pronouncements. Older parents whose offspring continued to live at home were increasingly faced with the question of how to make provision in the event of their own increasing frailty (Sanctuary, 1981). There were also, however, some developments in this period, which impacted on families' approaches and aspirations. As discussed in Chapter 2, normalisation theories began to influence policy and also enabled families to have different and higher expectations for their daughters and sons. This inevitably meant that battles with professionals continued as parents struggled to ensure that basic needs were met. Differences emerged, however, among parents' groups as to how this was to be achieved. Some families opposed institutional closure and focused on fund-raising to improve facilities in the hospitals; and some supported the idea of a safe, busy but still segregated lifestyle.

For others, an ordinary life now seemed to be within reach. And in some areas, a degree of collaboration between the Directors of some newly formed Social Services Departments and voluntary Societies meant that families were able to achieve changes. According to Michael Tombs:

> During my Chairmanship [of the Bedford Society], I remember being invited round to the Director's house and asked what should be the next project. I said 'A rural and horticultural day centre', and this happened and is still a successful project. (Rolph, 2005b, p. 59)

There were still tense moments, however, when the local authority was not moving as fast as the Society would have liked. Some parents spoke of their continuing crucial role as advocates. The ordinary life discourse was the precursor of a switch in emphasis by families to rights and citizenship on behalf of relatives with learning disabilities.

Experiments in education

Whereas in the early days of the Mencap Societies, parents did not on the whole challenge segregation, in this later period new ideas on inclusive services began to emerge, to be met with a mixed response from families, remaining a debating point today. As education had been the main catalyst for the founding of the first voluntary Societies in the 1940s and 1950s, so it became the focus for a shift in ideas of family roles and attitudes in the 1970s and 1980s. Some experiments in inclusive education were carried out by a Mencap Society in the 1970s and are an interesting example of the role of families in speaking out about local education policies. The Cambridge Mencap Society's Welfare Visitor responded to parents' worries about special education by setting up an Education Group (Rolph, 2005a). The Group's records show that parents 'shared their concerns, informed themselves of provisions and policies, and marshalled their ideas about future service provision'.[3] As a result, the Group began to speak for parents on issues such as integration, parental choice, parents as co-therapists and parents' roles in assessment. Significantly, it also set up an experimental unit (reminiscent of the Opportunity Classes) for children with learning difficulties in an independent school and provided the impetus for an Integration Group, a mixed group of professional workers and parents. In the experimental unit:

> Four of the children in the unit of six are Downs syndrome and two are slow learners: their ages range from five to ten years. They have their own 'specialist trained' teacher in the mornings, and in the afternoons they either join in the normal reception class or they go to the city Sports Hall for trampolining and gym.[4]

Despite these experiments and later developments in inclusive education, there are divisions in the parents' movement, and tensions remain high between those who advocate integration and those families who, as a result of bad experiences or because of strongly held views or generational differences, still maintain the right to segregated services for their offspring.

The rights agenda gained further impetus in 1984 when the first self-advocacy group – London People First – was set up. This provided a challenge for some families who had been used to advocating *for* their children for many years, and tensions remain between some families and the self-advocacy movement (Mitchell, 1999). The movement began to take on the role previously held by parents. Many families have acknowledged that though their campaigning role continues, this role has now been taken up independently by their offspring who are also campaigning for change on their own behalf.

Gestures towards families' incorporation into policymaking mean that they are now formally, if not necessarily meaningfully, part of the policy-making process. Despite this, and the work done by families to try to gain a foothold in forums influential in policy change, families feel they still have to be vigilant in the face of continuing discrimination and prejudice. Parents continue to be given misinformation by the medical profession or are refused treatment for their children, and families report that services are being withdrawn under the banner of independence and citizenship (Concannon, 2004). They are distrustful of changes – and in particular fear the seemingly enforced moves from one group home to another and the closure of the Day Centres. One parent said:

> There is still much to be done. Clearly we need to be working towards the time when the lives of people with learning disabilities will more closely parallel those of their siblings, with relatively smooth transitions at each of the milestones along the way from childhood to adulthood. (Crabbe in Rolph, 2005a)

At the same time, families from black and minority ethnic groups are speaking up about double discrimination and their social exclusion because of racism (Baxter *et al.*, 1990; Mir *et al.*, 2001).

There are also more positive testimonies, however, which indicate that the Societies' stated role of 'watchdog' has borne fruit in some areas and that there is now a greater awareness and understanding among the general public, as well as greater opportunities for people with learning difficulties: 'I see a lot more parents walking their children to ordinary schools, and buildings getting changed'(Monck in Rolph *et al.*, 2005, p. 329). Some parents are convinced that the startling changes in opportunities, choices and rights, together with access to independent life-styles, housing, and other types of supported accommodation, are due in large part to the determined campaigning of families over the past half century, either individually, or collectively in the voluntary Societies. What is believed by many, however, is that these improvements and gains are not necessarily secure and unchanging. The fact that so many of the same battles and struggles recur in each period is an indication that the role of vigilant campaigner cannot safely be relinquished.

Conclusion

The parents' role as advocates for their sons and daughters is a strand that links family stories over the decades from 1948. The central role of families is the one constant in the many vicissitudes in the history of community control and care. It is difficult to claim that families changed policy. And yet, they aimed and campaigned to do so, and there are important examples of progress being made at a local level because of the intervention of families and voluntary Societies. The oral history testimonies of families, set alongside government White Papers and legislation, suggest that it is clear that, despite changes in government attitude and intention, the policy often disappointed. One major change has occurred: in arguing initially for specialist provision and latterly for inclusion in mainstream education, occupational and living opportunities, many (though by no means all) parents have increasingly adopted the language of rights and citizenship. The parental discourse of citizenship – and all the rights that go with this – has in turn been adopted in the policy documents, particularly in *Valuing People*. And families as carers were for the first time included in its preparation. Families have both influenced the shift from control to care to citizenship and, at the same time, have been influenced by it, though as the stories by parents in this chapter have shown, there has been no Whiggish march of progress, but a hesitant and circular trail: continuity as well as change.

Notes

1. Bedford LEA to Brenda Nickson, September 1959.
2. Interview with the author, 2001.
3. Cambridgeshire Collection, Cambridge (hereafter CC): Cambridge Mencap Society Archive.
4. CC: *Cambridge Year Book, 1979/80*.

12

In the Shadow of the Poor Law: Workforce Issues

Duncan Mitchell and John Welshman

Introduction

Alan Bennett's *Untold Stories* (2005) opens with a vignette of discussions between Bennett, his father, and Mr Parr, the MWO. These took place in September 1966, in Settle, North Yorkshire, and concerned Bennett's mother, who had been admitted to the Lancaster Moor Hospital, suffering from delusions (Bennett, 2005, p. 3). The description is a rare one, of discussions between a family and a representative of statutory services. Moreover it is illustrative of how the 1960s has often been seen in terms of mental health rather than learning disability. MWOs dealt with both mental health and learning disability, but the two were often combined in policy documents, and, as today, it was often the former that assumed precedence over the latter. Key to the well-being of people with learning difficulties is the quality and commitment of the people who work with them. This is true whether people live in institutions or in their own homes in the community. Yet attention to the workforce has been extremely low profile in policy initiatives. Despite community care being a reality for several decades for a large number of people, there has not been a substantial investment in developing a workforce which is fit for the new roles community living requires.

Previous chapters have demonstrated the complexity of community care, and this can be further illustrated by the workforce in community services. In examining the learning disability workforce, we will be considering the roles that different occupational groups have played in relation to care, control and rights. Perhaps because there has been no strategic attention paid to the workforce, unlike in Australia, (see Chapter 9) an enormously wide range of staff groups have been part of the history of care in the community. These include staff in Occupation

Centres and hostels, DAOs and MWOs, social workers, psychiatrists, psychologists, GPs, nurses, home teachers, foster carers and small home residential care staff. Since more people now live 'in the community' this list stretches even further to include service personnel in a wide range of industries. The history of the relationship between people with learning disabilities and staff has yet to be properly explored. The history of staff and the development of services has fared a little better, but is still far from comprehensive, apart from work on learning disability nurses; a study of MWOs in East Anglia; and some work on the wardens of hostels (Mitchell, 2000; Rolph *et al.*, 2002, 2003; Welshman, 2006a). This chapter discusses the various categories of staff involved in the care of people with learning disabilities, but it also explores broader themes – difficulties in defining the nature of the work; the poor value accorded to much of it; the inappropriate models of care in which many staff have had to work; and an ideological ambivalence about the nature of staff alongside their motivation and remuneration. As with the other chapters in Part IV, it uses a mix of documentary and oral sources.

An overview of workforce issues, 1948–2001

In 2001, there were an estimated 83,000 people in the learning disability workforce, 33,000 in local authorities, 30,000 in the voluntary and independent sectors and 20,000 in the NHS. However around 75 per cent of these were unqualified (DOH, 2001a, p. 96). The postwar failure to properly address the issue of location of services was compounded by a failure to develop an adequate staffing policy for the service. In the absence of a consensus about the needs of the service, the Government effectively allowed the staffing practices of the prewar service to develop in a haphazard way. This meant that the models adopted by the wider mental health services were used for the development of staffing the mental deficiency services. The result was that although there were community services, these can only be understood within the context of the shadow of the institutions that continued to grow until reaching a static figure of just over 58,000 patients from 1954 (DHSS, 1971, p. 18). When reform was proposed in the early 1970s, staff development was hampered as energies were put into improving practices within the institutions at the cost of developing people to work within community settings (Townsend, 1969; Jones, 1975).

It is certainly clear that there has been a consistent problem in turnover of staff within learning disability services (Rose, 1995). This has been the case for all staff, but qualified staff have been particularly difficult to recruit. *Better Services* was clear that the 'shortage of staff, particularly trained staff, is a limiting factor to the quality and further development of every part of the local authority services' (DHSS, 1971, p. 17). It went on to detail shortages among social workers, and staff of ATCs, as well as residential homes. The problem was particularly acute amongst trained staff and the White Paper acknowledged the dearth of opportunities for training for local authority work in this area. At the end of our period, *Valuing People* perceived the main problems and challenges in workforce training and planning as being: difficulties in recruitment and retention, low status, a lack of recognised training qualifications, little attention to workforce planning and variable involvement of service users and carers in training or planning (DOH, 2001a, p. 96).

Prior to 1948, paid staff had been employed by local authorities and voluntary organisations. The NHS took over the organisation of the majority of the large institutional provision and in so doing created a third employer. The learning disability workforce was now employed by local authorities, the NHS and voluntary organisations. Workers in learning disability services were an afterthought in service reconfigurations and had to fit in with structures designed to meet the needs of acute hospital and mental health services. The largest groups of qualified workers were nurses, MWOs and instructors and teachers. Other professional workers such as GPs had an important role to play but were not specialists in learning disability. Psychiatrists who, as Medical Superintendents of the institutions, had considerable power were also significant players in the service. Alongside the professional workers was a much larger group of unqualified staff who, together with many people with learning disabilities, did much of the work involved in maintaining the various services. Residential staff, other than a small proportion of those working in hospitals, were not required to be qualified although some had been trained in previous work (Jones, 1975). Other residential staff were employed by local authorities or voluntary organisations.

This position remained largely the same until the reorganisation of services in the early 1970s consolidated the partial division between health and Social Services by creating a generic social work profession employed entirely by Social Services. From this point, the workforce for people with learning disabilities was organised into community care by Social Services and large institutional care by the NHS. This division began to break down as hospitals began to resettle people into NHS-run community services and to employ both residential staff and community learning disability nurses in the late 1970s, and as the private and voluntary sectors began to run services. By 2001, there remained a professional workforce numerically dominated by nurses and social workers, and a much larger unqualified workforce employed by health, local authorities and private and voluntary organisations. The position had changed a great deal since 1948. The long-stay institutions that had flourished in the 1950s and 1960s were mostly closed by 2001, and the vast majority of staff working with people with learning disabilities did so in community settings. Despite this evident change, there are some constant themes in the history of staffing learning disability services between 1948 and 2001.

The importance of staff: the views of service users

Autobiographical and biographical accounts of the lives of people with learning disabilities demonstrate a very mixed picture of the staff involved in the lives of individuals. Mabel Cooper, for example, explains how a particular member of staff helps her:

> Mary is my carer now. She buys the clothes for me because I find that's difficult. Mary does it for me because my eyesight's not that brilliant and the writing's so small. I can't read the labels so Mary does it. Jean lives at Mary's, she's all right, she helped me write a letter last night. She can't walk very much but otherwise she's okay. So I've got Jean and I've got Mary, so there is people there. (Cooper, 1997, p. 31)

However Cooper also tells different stories of staff who were oppressive and judgemental (Cooper, 2000). There are many such examples, and excerpts from the lives of people with learning disabilities can be used to demonstrate both negative and positive practice by individual members of staff within a variety of models of services. It is clear that staff have had significant power to individually affect the lives of people with learning disabilities but can only be one element in improving services, albeit a crucial one.

Duly Authorised Officers (DAOs) and Mental Welfare Officers (MWOs)

The legacy of the past and its impact on both hospital and community services has already been discussed. However difficulties in relation to this legacy have been compounded by the continuation of inappropriate models of care, even when settings have changed. Members of staff, sometimes individually and sometimes collectively, often retained practices from previous, or individually preferred, models of care. This often made change difficult as habits and attitudes became entrenched. The introduction of the NHS and local authority mental health services saw the creation of a new cadre of staff, MWOs, charged with supervision of care in the community (Means and Smith, 1994; Bartlett and Wright, 1999). In the late 1940s, the Ministry of Health turned to the DAOs, who were largely recruited from an existing group, the Poor Law Relieving Officers (ROs). The ROs had been 'duly authorised' under the 1890 Lunacy Act to be responsible for certification and for the compulsory admissions of 'pauper lunatics'. The DAOs had two main roles: compulsory hospital admissions for psychiatric cases and a supporting role in community care. Their main tasks for people with learning disabilities were in terms of doing statutory visits, monitoring and surveillance in the community, in order to control lives, with removal to hospital if families were thought unfit to care for and control their relatives (Rolph *et al.*, 2002, p. 32).

Much of the day-to-day activity of local authority personnel was in list making. The DAOs kept lists of the number of 'mental defectives' that had been 'dealt with'. Cases were classified under the Mental Deficiency Acts as being statutory, voluntary, guardianship, miscellaneous or 'friendly observation'. Under the arrangements under Section 28 of the NHS Act, lists were also made of those visited at home by Aftercare and Investigation Officers. Some of the concerns evident in the 1920s about sexuality and pregnancy were still evident in the case notes of people on licence, and in guardianship orders, in the 1940s (Walmsley *et al.*, 1999, p. 196). DAOs and MWOs were predominantly male, further indicating that their job was anticipated as being one of control rather than care; speedy removal to hospital, rather than casework support at home (Rolph *et al.*, 2003, p. 355).

The hospitals themselves were a visible and enduring presence of institutional care, and staff working in the community also lived with the legacy of the Poor Law. Earlier work has suggested that there were strong continuities between the old Public Assistance ROs and the supposedly new MWOs, and this is borne out by sources at the local level. In Lancashire, for example, many of the MWOs were former Poor Law ROs, illustrating further continuities with the pre-NHS era (Jones, 1954, pp. 39–47). The same applied in Bedfordshire (French, 1972). The Younghusband Report on social work, for example, noted that there was no recognised qualification for Welfare Officers. Since 1948, appointments had been made in the light of knowledge, experience as a RO and a general aptitude for the work; 40 per cent held qualifications, usually (in England and Wales) the RO's Certificate (Ministry of Health, 1959, pp. 84–90). Studies of care in the community by social scientists provided further insights into the experience and qualifications of MWOs. A case study of Manchester found that male MWOs were ex-ROs employed by the Board of Guardians, while their female equivalents were unqualified (Rodgers and Dixon, 1960, pp. 45–50).

Oral evidence demonstrates that MWOs were not always clear about their roles, and visits sometimes became habitual. One former MWO paid routine visits to a mother and her son J who lived in a remote Norfolk village:

> I used to pop in as part of the mental deficiency list, just spoke to Mrs So and So, 'Is he alright?' He'd hide away or he'd be down the garden, but he actually got to know me and he'd come to the garden gate to see me off ... over the years I got to know him. The doctor who had been looking after that village for years just accepted them as they were, they didn't want to be interfered with, nothing was ever done for him, nothing was ever wanted. (Rolph *et al.*, 2003, p. 345)

This is an interesting account of benign visiting. The family may have been afraid that the MWO would take J away as would have been possible under the Mental Deficiency Act, and the work of the MWO therefore ensured that some contact was maintained even if the individual visits had little purpose. For some, however, the visits became more punitive as Neville Porter recounts:

> When they [mental defectives] were on licence you used to visit them fairly regularly, quite often. I mean in those days you used to handle the odd 'moral defective'. A girl who had a baby was ostracised in the village, used to finish up in the Hospital [for people with learning difficulties] ... you know, never ought to have been there and it was very difficult for them to be discharged (Rolph *et al.*, 2003, p. 346).

Training did improve, and some MWOs were offered places on nurse training courses in hospitals. Overall, the way that DAOs and MWOs perceived their role provides an illuminating perspective on the development of services for people with learning difficulties, especially in the period up to 1971.

Workforce issues at the local authority level, 1948–71

Apart from the MWOs, a range of staff were employed by local authorities, and these included social workers, those who helped to run JTCs and

ATCs, and the wardens of local hostels. The MWOs were able to advocate on behalf of their clients, by making a case for home support and by supporting parents' groups, and they also undertook casework and social work with families, to avert admission or prevent re-admission to hospital (Rolph *et al.*, 2003, p. 357). Some MWOs were moving towards a closer relationship with social workers, in those areas that had appointed them. Their role in augmenting community facilities such as developing clubs, lodgings and jobs ran parallel to a growing involvement in aftercare and casework, and a growing identity as social workers. Furthermore, some local authorities recruited from voluntary Mental Welfare Associations whose members were mostly women, and these workers were more likely to be concerned about bringing mental welfare work in line with professional social work practice (Rolph *et al.*, 2002, p. 37). Overall then, mental welfare work was heavily gendered, but there was an awareness that it would benefit from a move away from a medical or procedural focus, towards a closer relationship with the developing social work profession.

The Mackintosh Committee (1951) had argued that more psychiatric social workers were needed – 1500 instead of the 331 then in practice. An unpublished interim report (1949) had made recommendations on supply and demand, and on the training and goals of psychiatric social workers. More generally it encouraged the recruitment of men, advocated economies in trained staff and recommended the use of part-time workers (Ministry of Health, 1951, pp. 46–9). Nevertheless there is little evidence that the shortage of social workers was remedied. When the Younghusband Committee reported in 1959, it noted of the report of the Mackintosh Committee that 'seven years later, we can but echo many of the findings' (Ministry of Health, 1959, p. 52). There was still a large unfulfilled demand for social workers in the mental health services; a handful of psychiatric social workers in relation to demand; and still no training for other MWOs. This was all the more serious as the scope of the services, and the needs to be met, had grown as the Mackintosh Committee had foreseen.

The Younghusband Committee found that Welfare Officers and MWOs were working as social workers, and the Committee estimated that there were 1619 in total, of whom 625 worked entirely in the mental health services. Of these, 20 per cent were over 60 years of age, and 45 per cent were over 50 (Ministry of Health, 1959, pp. 84–90). Richard Titmuss argued on the publication of the Younghusband Report that 'large sections of the Mental Health Bill, now before Parliament, are pure fantasy without the trained staff to operate effective domiciliary services' (Titmuss, 1959, p. 11). The number of psychiatric social workers employed full-time by local authorities had only increased from 8 in 1951 to 26 in 1959. In 1961, Titmuss famously warned that:

> at present, we are drifting into a situation in which, by shifting the emphasis from the institution to the community – a trend which in principle and with qualifications we all applaud – we are transferring the care of the mentally ill from trained staff to untrained or ill-equipped staff or no staff at all. (Titmuss, 1961, p. 356)

While Titmuss chose to use mental health as his example, his point was equally applicable to learning disability. The *Health and Welfare* White Paper revealed that local authorities employed only 1128 social workers (0.024 per 1000 population), again raising the question of what the slow development of services meant for individual families (Ministry of Health, 1963, pp. 24–30).

Social work was an important influence on the Seebohm Report (1968). There had occurred a rapid increase in the numbers of social workers in the 1960s, with the number in the mental health services increasing, to 1808 in 1969 (Moroney, 1976, pp. 79–82), and the Seebohm Report illustrated the effectiveness of the social work profession as a lobbying group. The creation of Social Services Departments marked a victory for social work over the rival claims of public health (DHSS, 1968, p. 108). It led to the incorporation of MWOs into a generic social work profession (DHSS, 1968). Whilst some social workers continued to specialise in learning disabilities, it was the end of a separate mental health part of the social work profession. Nevertheless important rivalries at the local level continued to impede the development of services. Kathleen Jones found from her study that contacts with Social Services Departments were generally good but that wardens of hostels did not want social workers to visit 'their' residents too often and found them liable to 'interfere' (Jones, 1975, p. 177).

As we saw in Chapter 3, the Seebohm Report made recommendations affecting responsibility for ATCs and JTCs. Educational and instructional staff employed in both JTCs and ATCs, if qualified, were trained through the NAMH training scheme and were employed by local authorities or a small number of voluntary organisations. The qualification for Training Centre staff was the Diploma of the Training Council for Teachers of the Mentally Handicapped. But in fact Kathleen Jones found in her survey that only 30 per cent of all staff were qualified, and of the ten authorities with Training Centres she investigated, three had no qualified staff at all. There was an acute shortage of staff, whether trained or untrained. The official staff–trainee ratio was 1:15, but in most of the Centres, the ratio was 1:18 or 1:20 (Jones, 1975, p. 164). She found that in ATCs, staff–trainee relationships were often of a very limited kind, based on staff authoritarianism and the maintenance of social distance. Male trainees often addressed staff as 'sir', and staff clearly saw their role as a supervisory one, based on the need for increased productivity, rather than as therapy or education (Jones, 1975, p. 165). This relates to the wider issue of work, discussed in Chapters 1 and 3.

As care in the community gradually expanded, including the opening of hostels at the local level, the qualifications, performance and aptitude of the personnel who staffed them came under increasing scrutiny. In the case of hostels, the key member of staff was the warden. In his study of hostels for the mentally ill, Robert Apte found that MOsH saw wardens as parental figures; as people who could help residents find employment or conform to the 'standards of the community' (Apte, 1968, p. 43). Nevertheless there was no recognised training for wardens, and while half of the wardens had qualifications in nursing, half had no relevant training beyond secondary school. Three-quarters had worked in medical or non-medical institutions, and brought values and modes of behaviour typical of institutional environments. This limited the extent to which the hostels could encourage rehabilitation (Apte, 1968, p. 113). Studies of wardens in other types of residential settings, such as probation hostels, found that hostels were like families, and the influence of the warden and the matron analogous to that of parents. Hostels were dependant on the warden and matron; parental qualities were demanded of these members of staff; and staff and residents had a high degree of interdependence (Sinclair, 1975, p. 136).

Wardens were of course also needed to staff hostels for people with learning disabilities. Like Apte, Kathleen Jones found that a great deal depended on the personalities and attitudes of the wardens in hostels, and while some had nursing qualifications, others had none, though most had institutional experience of some kind (Jones, 1975, pp. 175–6). Jones found one Deputy Warden, an ex-prison officer, wore a white coat, and spent part of his time while on duty sitting at the reception desk in the hall; in another, the warden, formerly a hospital sister, insisted on being called 'matron' (Jones, 1975, p. 176). Staff have had a great deal of power to influence the ways that people live their lives; this has sometimes transcended organisational culture as individual staff have been able to apply their own views and attitudes to their work. Jones, for example, observed that the atmosphere and activities within hostels depended on the views and energy of the wardens. Some organised birthday parties, games and competitions, but others took the view that this sort of organisation bore the marks of institutionalisation, and that residents were far happier spending their spare time as they pleased, watching television, chatting or staying in their own rooms (Jones, 1975, p. 175). However because of their obvious care and concern for the well-being of residents, most hostels were warm, friendly places in which the majority of residents could feel at home (Jones, 1975, p. 176; Welshman, 2006a). In these ways staff can have a positive or negative effect on people with learning disabilities.

The difficulty in defining what was required of workers in learning disability services reflected a wider confusion about the services themselves. Although there was a growing consensus about the need to close hospitals from the 1970s, there was less agreement about what was to replace them. Local decision making led to many different patterns of care needing varying types of workers. This, combined with the inadequate provision of services for people who had never lived in institutions, led to a widely disparate picture in which a number of agencies with different models of paid work organised services in local areas. Such lack of consistency did not help to add value to a workforce already demoralised by hospital scandals, poor conditions and low pay. Indeed there is evidence that work with people with learning disabilities has been undervalued within professions as well as from outside (Mitchell, 2000). When this is combined with the poor value attached to domestic and caring work in other areas, then it is not surprising that work with people with learning disabilities has suffered from poor recruitment. There have been attempts to avoid such transfer of behaviours from one model of care to another. Some resettlement schemes for example avoided employing staff with previous experience of hospital work, while warning of the pitfalls of employing untrained and inexperienced staff.

Learning disability nursing

In 1948, the NHS was divided into hospital and community services. The former were responsible for the large learning disability institutions and employed Medical Superintendents (with various deputies) and nursing staff to run them. The implementation of this arrangement led to the further development of a nursing workforce based largely on general hospital models. Most nursing staff remained unqualified. Whilst some nurses moved into work with people with learning disabilities outside the institutions, for the majority their work took place exclusively within them. Nursing followed a different path to social work with the Briggs Committee recommending that a separate profession evolve to work with people with learning disabilities with the Jay Committee confirming this (*Report of the Committee of Enquiry*, 1979). Despite these reports, learning disability nursing remained a separate part of nursing and increasingly transferred its work from institutional to community services.

There was a question about the nature of nursing work with people with learning disabilities: were they involved in the care of the sick or the training and development of healthy people? (Mitchell, 2000). There was also a wider question about the activities that staff were to be required to carry out in a reformed service. The 1971 White Paper tried to achieve reform within the hospitals as well as development of services outside them, but it did imply that staff wanted change. It acknowledged that 'very few [hospitals] have had the resources to do anything like as much as the staff themselves want to do' (DHSS, 1971, p. 20). Kathleen Jones argued that the persistence of the 'medical' model of treatment meant there were large numbers of people called 'doctors' and 'nurses' whose work did not primarily involve the medical and nursing skills in which they had been trained, while other people who had the necessary skills were either not employed at all or employed in very small numbers and relegated to a subordinate position where their work was only minimally effective (Jones, 1975, p. 97).

This in part reflects previous debates that have questioned the value of professional training. The Jay Committee drew attention to this issue but concluded that training was not in itself a barrier to being a satisfactory worker. It tried to put staff at the centre of service development by turning a Committee that was set up to look into mental handicap nursing and care into one that recommended a new blueprint for services by arguing that 'it would be impossible to examine care and the training and deployment of staff without looking at complementary issues of setting, organisation and resources' (*Report of the Committee of Inquiry*, 1979, p. 1). However there were tensions. The Jay Committee believed that the 'naturalness and spontaneity of the residential care worker' could be left intact by training and that the additional knowledge, skills, sensibilities and intelligent thought which good training brought could help to create a caring person who would be nurtured by improved models of residential care (*Report of the Committee of Enquiry*, 1979, p. 53). The reforms of the 1970s may have begun to achieve consensus about hospital closure and the development of community services, but this did not lead to a consensus about the work of the staff, even of staff working in specific areas such as residential care. According to the Jay Report, for example, 'those who gave evidence to us found it hard to express what the tasks of the residential care worker consisted of, except in very broad terms' (*Report of the Committee of Enquiry*, 1979, p. 52). This conclusion may have influenced the Government in its decision to retain learning disability nursing despite the recommendations of both the Jay and Briggs Reports. Nursing came from a background model of care that seemed totally unsuitable for community services for people with learning disabilities but the Government, possibly recognising the ability to change and adapt, did not agree. It stated that it was not the time to abandon a well-tried form of training for nurses – who would continue to provide the majority of mental handicap care staff – for one which was comparatively new and vigorously opposed by nurses and major voluntary organisations.[1] The result was a number of educational schemes that were designed to combine the social and nursing models of care with a clear intention of using the education of staff to change services. A review of the 1971 White Paper published in 1980 indicated that specialist services were still in their infancy, and that because there had been no central guidance there were a variety of approaches (DHSS, 1980). This, combined with the development of many different schemes for the resettlement of people from long-stay institutions, led to a confused pattern. The House of Commons Select Committee on Social Services (1985) argued that qualified Community Mental Handicap Nurses should not be used simply as additional residential care staff. Caring for mentally handicapped people did not require skills which were the exclusive preserve of nurses; distinctive nursing skills were required in some circumstances, but the basic tending, social care or educative skills could also be deployed by other professionals (House of Commons, 1985, section 198).

Later attempts at joint training in the 1990s combined nursing and social work at undergraduate level and had some success although they continued to have difficulties in combining different models based on health and social care (Fagan and Plant, 2003). There is clearly a tension between normal patterns of living and paid care. It is difficult to have the former without the latter, but nevertheless paid care itself is less likely to be valued than full independence. There have also been tensions between advocates of specialist and generic services. For example deinstitutionalisation has been accompanied by an emphasis on enabling people with learning difficulties to access mainstream services for their health care, transport and leisure. This creates the need for a very wide range of workers to have some awareness of the particular challenges people with learning difficulties face, and training as a means to communicate with them. However people meet doctors and other health care professionals who fail to offer appropriate health care; bus drivers who lack patience and fail to deter name calling and bullying; police who dismiss reports of crimes; and countless other groups of employees who lack the understanding that this group has particular needs.

Conclusion

This chapter has explored the history of staff who worked in institutions and community services for people with learning disabilities. The reality is that paid staff are fundamentally a part of a system and have their own interests, such as pay and conditions that are sometimes at variance from the needs of people with learning difficulties. There is also ambivalence within staff groups themselves. Staff have played important roles in closing the institutions yet, at the same time, some of the main opposition to institutional closure came from organisations representing the workforce (Oswin, 2000). There is a belief, fostered in particular by SRV, that people who are motivated by commitment, rather than cash or status, are the ones who are needed. This is demonstrated sharply by the roles of self advocacy support workers, who lack recognised training, career development opportunities and adequate remuneration, yet are expected to carry out the extremely delicate task of supporting individuals to speak out, at the same time as helping self-advocates raise cash, fulfil contracts and generally run a business (Chapman, 2005). Similar arguments apply to volunteer advocates. There is resistance to making payments to them, and to imposing a code of conduct, yet it is an extremely difficult and demanding role (Atkinson, 1999).

Some of the themes that have been highlighted in this chapter are the continuities in personnel between the Poor Law and the early NHS; the considerable freedom that some workers, such as wardens, had in interpreting their role, for good or for bad; the fact that trained workers, such as social workers remained relatively few in numbers into the 1960s; and the broader significance of training for rehabilitation and work, as was the case with the ATCs. The majority of staff working with people with learning difficulties have been untrained and unqualified. Although there have been initiatives to develop skills within the workforce (e.g., the target set in *Valuing People* for 50 per cent of front line staff to have achieved at least National Vocational Qualifications Level 2 by 2005)

(DOH, 2001a, p. 129), there have been several factors which have impeded the development of coherent career pathways for people specialising in learning disability. Ideas about 'progressive' services have been hampered by a failure to address issues of staff training and remuneration, and this is as true today as it was in the late 1950s, with massive staff turnover impacting on quality of life and services (Concannon, 2004). For example *Valuing People* suggests that staff commitment has only been able to go so far: 'despite the efforts of some highly committed staff, public services have failed to make consistent progress in overcoming the social exclusion of people with learning disabilities' (DOH, 2001a, p. 19). Whilst staff have been powerful in relation to people with learning disabilities, their power to influence service development has only been partial.

Note

1. DHSS, 1980, press release 80/189.

13
Implementation of Community Care: Case Studies

Dorothy Atkinson and Sheena Rolph

Introduction

In this chapter we consider community care in Croydon, an urban authority, and Norfolk, a predominantly rural county. The Croydon case study traces the implementation of community care through the lives and experiences of four women. The Norfolk case study interweaves the main narrative with the stories of six people with learning difficulties. Three themes are traced in both: education, living arrangements, and work/daytime occupation – echoing the themes of Chapter 3. This enables consideration of the impact of community care on how people lived and how they spent their time. There were connections between Croydon and Norfolk, part of the continuing migration of people with learning difficulties which had begun in the early part of the century (Rolph, 1999). Croydon residents were sometimes moved to residential placements in Norfolk and then returned when accommodation became available.

Croydon: Background

Croydon is an urban centre bordering London and adjoining the rural county of Surrey. Its location has helped determine the destinies of many people – some its own residents, others from elsewhere who were later resettled into Croydon from St Lawrence's Hospital. St Lawrence's was in nearby Caterham and was the legacy of the Victorian Metropolitan Asylums Board. It was a barrack-like institution housing around 2000 people. Although in many ways the antithesis of community care, it provided an *impetus* for community provision. In the absence of local authority services, it set up its own hostels: Chaldon

Mead, established in the 1930s for men and, in the 1950s, Whyteleafe House for women. The aim was to provide accommodation for people thought capable of holding down jobs. As Government policies switched to community care, the local authority began to provide services. The presence of a large institutional population on Croydon's doorstep provided a boost to development. Although St Lawrence's was opened in 1870, it became part of Croydon's story only after the 1946 NHS Act. Prior to that, people from Croydon thought to need institutional care were sent elsewhere: 'cases requiring this kind of treatment are sent to Institutions maintained by other local authorities'.[1] It had no institution of its own. Destinations included Botley's Park (Surrey County Council) and Cell Barnes (Hertfordshire County Council). Other children and adults were boarded out, for example, in Brighton under the supervision of the Brighton Guardianship Society.

Croydon lacked adequate day care. The sole prewar Occupation Centre was closed for the War and was subsequently considered unsuitable for re-opening. A new Occupation Centre opened in May 1948 with 8 children. A year later, 33 children, and by 1951, 43 children attended, with a waiting list of '20 cases'.[2] The shift to community care came particularly in the wake of the 1959 Mental Health Act, and similar patterns have been reported in Leicester and Bedfordshire (French, 1972; Welshman, 2000). Croydon saw the opening of Waylands and Cherry Orchard ATCs in the 1960s, Heaver's Farm in 1974, together with the Crosfield industrial and sheltered workshop complex, regarded at the time as 'an important scheme of industrial and social training' (Clarke and Clarke, 1972, p. 259). A three-tier system of ATC, Advanced ATC and sheltered workshop was established (Morley, 1973), aiming to place people in open or sheltered employment. The use of boarding out-schemes continued, later becoming the Social Services-run Adult Placement Scheme (APS). In 1963 eight people were boarded out in lodgings and 13 in foster homes supervised by the Brighton Guardianship Society.[3] From the 1980s, more diverse residential schemes developed, including private residential homes, hostels and bedsits, a pattern of provision which persisted.

The lived experience: the lives of four women

The account so far has come from documentary sources. The story is now told through the testimonies of four women who experienced the changes. Table 2 summarises their biographical details. In childhood, three were separated from their families. This marked the beginning of segregation and eventually led each to admission to St Lawrence's. Mary Coventry, by contrast, was educated locally and continued to live with her parents well into adulthood.

The table shows change beginning in the 1960s, when social workers began to find outside employment for Doris Thorne. Some were day jobs from the hospital, some were live-in posts, and others saw her boarded-out with landladies and families. Lack of support meant that many were short-lived and ended in her return to hospital. Doris recalled work in a laundry in the 1960s:

> I worked years ago in a laundry on St James's Road in Croydon. I worked as a shirt-presser. That was all right, I got a good report. I only lost my temper once, and that was because I had to do a special shirt for a gentleman. It kept coming out creased ... I was living in St Lawrence's then, and had to catch a bus at half past five. I started early. I had to be there by seven. (Thorne, 2005)

The early start, long days, and hard work took their toll. Many jobs followed, including this one in the 1970s:

> I was a domestic at the hotel, and I also worked in the kitchen. It was heavy work; I had big pots and pans to wash. I lived there as well, I was there for $9^1/_2$ weeks. There was always arguments, carries on – terrible it was. The staff when they came in never said 'Good morning, Doris' ... Nobody would talk to you ... it ended with me crying. The boss said I had to go before anyone else goes. (Thorne, 2005)

In the 1970s, Gloria, Mabel and Doris were placed in Whyteleafe house. It was intended to provide for women what Chaldon Mead had offered men since 1931: 'These two hostels played an important role in return-ing suitable patients to outside life; "they're valuable stepping stones to residence outside the community", as the Board of Control visitors said in 1959' (Malster, 1994, p. 72). Whyteleafe House worked for Gloria and Mabel, but not for Doris who stayed only a short time before returning to St Lawrence's. Mabel describes it a continuation of St Lawrence's:

> Whyteleafe House was the same as St Lawrence's, the only difference is that it was a house. It was still a big place. It was no different because they still had nurses and what-have-you. You still had 50 people. It was all women. I shared a room with six others. Whyteleafe House used to be for people what used to go out to work, they didn't take

Table 2 Biographical summaries (Croydon)

Year	Gloria Ferris (b. 1939)	Doris Thorne (b. 1941)	Mabel Cooper (b. 1944)	Mary Coventry (b. 1944)
1940	1941: Fountain Hospital 1940s: Special School from hospital	1940s: Local Special School	1940s: Residential nursery and children's homes	1940s: At home with parents and brother
1950	1952: Residential school 1956: St Lawrence's Meets Muriel	1950s: Residential Special School (Birmingham) 1955: St Lawrence's	1950s: Children's homes and residential school 1955: St Lawrence's	1950s: Private primary (day) school, then local Special School
1960	1960s: Nursing and domestic work (unpaid) at St Lawrence's	1960s: Laundry, factory and domestic work – from hospital (some as live-in jobs)	1960s: Living in hospital	1960s: Social Services Department-run Day Centres (living in the family home)
1970	1972: Whyteleafe House – local domestic work 1970s: Live-in domestic work at Purley Hospital	1970s: Whyteleafe House 1970s: Factory and domestic work – from hospital (some as live-in jobs)	1970s: Whyteleafe House Boarding-out placements in family homes 1970s: Domestic work, then unemployed	1970s: Attends Day Centre and lives in the family home

1980	1980s: Family home in APS. Domestic work in homes and hospitals 1988: Moves into (current) family home in APS	1980s: Moves from St Lawrence's to live with a foster family. Returns to hospital	1980s: Private home in APS. 1980s: People First, Croydon and London	1980s: Attends Day Centre 1980s: Part-time post as People First secretary 1986: Bedsit in group home
1990	1994: Made redundant. Foxley Lodge part-time (day care) 1990s: Joins Advocacy Partners; becomes Muriel's advocate and Advocacy Partners committee member	1990s: Moves to private home (small hostel) Acquires an advocate	1990s: Foxley Lodge (part-time) 1990s: Family home in APS. Continues People First work	1990s: Continues Day Centre, People First secretarial work and lives in the bedsit

anybody else. And then they said, 'Oh well, we haven't got enough people now what go out to work, we'll have to change it and put other people there' ... I lived at Whyteleafe House, they used to pick me up at the house and take me to the hospital for the day. At night-time they used to take me back. (Cooper, 1997, pp. 29–30)

Gloria's experience was more positive. She lived there and worked as a domestic in an older people's home. She went on to work as a live-in domestic at Purley Hospital. This sort of arrangement was not uncommon (Walmsley and Rolph, 2001). Doris, Mabel and Gloria were placed together again in the 1980s when they lived at Isabel's – a private home run by an ex-nurse from St Lawrence's. This started as a family concern, but as demand grew, Isabel's home expanded. Gloria recalled:

She didn't have many in those days, only three of us. Then it got too big, too many, and I decided I wanted to move and go to a smaller place. I asked Anne Evans who was my Adult Placement Officer in those days if I could leave Isabel's and go to another place. (Ferris, 1998)

Mabel also decided it had become too big and noisy. She and Gloria put in (separate) requests to the APS for a move. They were each placed with home carers under Croydon's boarding-out scheme which has survived as an alternative to residential care. Things got off to a good start for Gloria in 1988 when she met her prospective carer:

And then I saw this dog – they had a dog – and I thought, oh, I'd like that. She came to me straight away. Norah said they wanted somebody who didn't smoke and, of course, I don't smoke ... I've been there ever since. (Ferris, 1998)

Mabel moved in 1992 to live with Mary (also an ex-nurse):

I want to say about Mary, the lady I live with, because she's so good and so understanding ... Since I've been there she has helped me to do the things I can't do, like matching clothes up, like using the shower, like keeping calm so my face doesn't swell, and like reading, if she has time. (Cooper, 2000, p. 188)

After a spell with foster parents, Doris was part of the 'new wave' of people moving to Isabel's. She enjoyed it, and stayed throughout its expansion in the 1990s. Fostering has continued throughout the postwar period. The original fostering schemes, supervised by the Brighton Guardianship Society, were part of a system of control as well as 'care' in the community.

Mary Coventry lived with her parents until 1986. She knew about St Lawrence's. She remembered: 'My mum did say to me that if I didn't behave I'd go to St Lawrence's so fast my feet wouldn't touch the ground' (Coventry, 2000, p. 194). When she left school, Mary attended Day Centres, including Waylands, until it – and other Croydon Day Centres – faced closure following a Best Value review in 2000. In the mid-1980s Mary's parents made enquiries about residential care which led to admission to Northampton Road, a mixed group home where she has a bedsit. Mary recounts:

> I left home on 24 March 1986. My parents ... said if they died, if any-thing happened to them, they would like to know that I was being looked after. They wanted to get me settled while they were still alive, and I accepted it [...] I said, well, that would be nice. They said there wouldn't be anyone to look after me in Bradmore Way ... . (Coventry, 2000, pp. 195–6)

In the 1990s, Mabel and Gloria attended Foxley Lodge, a privately-run Day Centre for 22 people. Mabel regarded it as a 'great centre': 'They help us with things like knitting, sewing, cooking, telling us how much we weigh, reading and writing. It's quite small, and very nice' (Cooper, 2000, p. 188). A thread which now links their lives is advocacy. In the 1980s, Mabel joined People First in Croydon and later became the Chairperson. She later became the chairperson of London People First. Self-advocacy became her career until the 1990s when the publication of her life story found her in great demand as a speaker. Mary became secretary at Croydon People First, alongside her Day Centre place.

In 1994, Gloria became the 'registered advocate' for Muriel, whom she had met in St Lawrence's in the 1950s. She had kept in touch with Muriel for 20 years until she gained this recognition. Gloria 'speaks up for her':

> If you've got a tongue in your head to speak for yourself then you speak up. Like Muriel, she can't speak, so I speak for her and ask for the things that she needs done for her. That's what they call 'being an advocate'. (Ferris, 1998, p. 193)

Gloria is a committee member for Advocacy Partners and takes part in the selection and training of advocates – advocacy had become her career in later life. Doris had also benefited from the growth of advocacy. She acquired an advocate, support which has proved crucial in the final move (post 2001) from Isabel's to a bedsit in a (private) home for people with learning difficulties. Doris explains Jane's role:

> She helps me quite a lot. I met her at a club in South Croydon ... I've been friends with her ever since ... She was glad when I moved out of Russell Hill. She could only get to see me after 8 o'clock and when she came after eight, they rushed her out. She said to me, 'You're not staying here for much longer. We're going to get you somewhere else'. She spoke to Maxine [care manager], told her about it, that's how I got to move. (Thorne, 2005)

Summary

The biographies shed light on community care. Residential care in Croydon and district ranged from institutional care in St Lawrence's via the stepping-stone hostel (Whyteleafe) to a mixed economy of a boarding-out scheme alongside a network of private homes and bedsits. Daytime occupation ranged from unsupported open employment to council-run and private Day Centres and, latterly, advocacy. The user movement, through advocacy in its various forms, has had a profound impact, creating new opportunities in their later lives.

Norfolk: Background

Norfolk is a large rural county with an extensive seaboard with towns often isolated economically and socially from the rest of the county. The main city, Norwich, had its own Borough Council, as did Great Yarmouth and Kings Lynn. Norfolk County Council provides for a scattered population, with poor transport links. These factors – compounded by a lack of political will – resulted in slow implementation of Government policies and contrasting approaches by different local authorities. There was a history of early progress in local responses in Norfolk to the 1913 and 1927 Mental Deficiency Acts, followed by delays and disagreements between two major local authorities, Norfolk and Norwich. There was no large institution until 1930 and many people were sent out of county or to the Norwich Poor Law Institution (Rolph, 2000). Unlike other counties where the push for change came largely from the Board of Control (Walmsley, 1994; Thomson, 1998a), Norfolk saw pressure from local authority officers and county councillors who voiced concern over lack of care and control of mental defectives. The two authorities finally agreed to act, although they responded in different ways.

In 1930, Norfolk County Council opened, first, Little Plumstead Colony (later Hospital), a few miles outside Norwich, and second, in 1933, Heckingham Institution, (later Hales Hospital), a former workhouse. At the same time, Norwich Borough Council implemented a type of community care by opening Eaton Grange, a hostel for women, close to the city centre. On the same site was the earliest local authority-run Occupation Centre in the country, opened originally in 1923. Norwich was unusual in setting up its own hostel. There were three categories of hostels set up in the interwar period: those associated with institutions such as Chaldon Mead in Croydon; those run privately or by voluntary associations; and, less usually, those run by local authorities. Eugenic fears undoubtedly played a part in Norwich. The Lord Mayor was reported as saying, 'if the hostel cannot cure, may it be the means of preventing more from being brought into the world'.[4] Apart from Eaton Grange, there were three private Approved Homes in Norwich.[5] Otherwise, services to families were few. After the opening of Little Plumstead, people began to be placed in the institution, though many remained with their families, a few helped by the Occupation Centre. In 1946, Norfolk County Council reported that provision had increased, with the appointment of one psychiatric social worker and 17 DAOs. Their role was:

> to assist the Medical Superintendent of the hospitals and the Mental Deficiency Colony in the matter of obtaining reports on home conditions, the supervision of patients at home 'on trial' or 'on leave', in reports following the admission of cases to hospital and follow-up reports when patients are on leave or discharged.[6]

This illustrates the kind of community care provided in Norfolk. It was a supervisory service, emphasising control as much as care.

The creation of the NHS meant that Norwich Borough Council passed Eaton Grange to a Hospital Management Committee (HMC) under the East Anglian RHB. Families were visited by an Enquiry Officer and many 'defectives' were placed under guardianship or supervision. Responsibility to provide services to those who stayed with their families remained with local authorities. A feature Norfolk shared with Croydon was the close link between colony and hostel, the latter providing a route into the community for women under supervision or licensing orders

(Thomson, 1998a; Rolph, 2000; Walmsley and Rolph, 2001). When the HMC took over the running of both hospital and hostel, these links were strengthened. The HMC then bought Blofield Hall, which in 1951 became a hostel and half-way house for men. Links between hospital and community were facilitated by these hostels, and continued until Little Plumstead closed in 2005 (see also Chapter 3).

The implementation of community care

Both residential provision and day services grew only gradually in the second half of the twentieth century, hampered by the perceived difficulties of distance and isolation and the resulting cost implications. What this meant on the ground is told in the testimonies of six people (Table 3). Their stories cover the three themes – education, living arrangements and work/daytime occupation.

Education: Schools and Occupation Centres

Provision of education or occupation was a low priority in the immediate postwar period. A survey was carried out in 1947 to ascertain and classify 'mental defectives' in the community. As a result, two more Occupation Centres were opened in 1949, one in Sprowston, Norwich and one in Kings Lynn, each taking 25 children and adults, while the Great Yarmouth Occupation Centre re-opened after the War. Sprowston in particular, was reported to be flourishing:

> During the year [1951] the Council purchased a second hand piano, and this has proved a great asset. The handwork made at the centres is sold at Open Days and the quality of the work greatly impressed the parents. The children were taken by staff to the seaside for the day.[7]

Glowing official reports are not always borne out by the testimonies of people involved. According to Betty Colby who worked at the Great Yarmouth Centre, the facilities were poor:

> We couldn't do much ... There was horrible old rush matting on the floor, you know, it wasn't very nice in the church hall. We only had one little toilet right out the back. We had school dinners ... We had to eat in the same room and afterwards two of the bigger boys used to collect the big galvanised bath and we used to have to wash up in the

same room. The same towel was used for all the children. (Rolph, 2002, p. 13)

The local authority was loathe to spend money on Occupation Centres. In 1952 the MOH's report stated '... in this large rural county the cost of transport prohibits the provision of full-time centres for all suitable children'.[8]

Having started at village schools, Jean Andrews and Douglas Lanham were later excluded but obtained places at the newly opened Sidestrand Boarding School in 1954 and 1956, respectively. Jean gained a place as a refuge from her abusive father. She said: 'I felt safer in boarding school. I went there for protection'. She had mixed emotions about her time there:

I got whipped with the cane, the cane! for being a nuisance! ... The caning didn't worry me very much – but I just used to go through it. I used to get wrong for not doing writing properly. You see, I couldn't grasp it ... but they said I'd get better and better, which I have. (Jean, 2002, p. 206)

To address the problems of the scattered population, a Home Teacher was appointed in 1950, and fortnightly 'Day Occupation Centres' were organised in seven areas. This meant that 35 children met in supervised groups to learn handicraft work.[9] It was judged successful and a second home teacher was employed for West Norfolk. By 1953, 116 were receiving home teaching, 34 attending Occupation Centres.

This attention to rural and seaside areas was due in part to the initiative of the Home Visitor:

Many will recall the first home teacher who organised groups of children to be conveyed to various points in Norfolk – her shooting brake bulged from door to door with children and equipment, but she always exuded cheerfulness and encouragement. [10]

Other rural counties made similar provision (Walmsley, 1994). After the 1959 Mental Health Act, Occupation Centres became JTCs, and several more were built. Oral testimony suggests little else changed. Stella Gill, a parent, described Norwich Occupation Centre:

It was a horrific place, Dickensian. The facilities were awful ... It was a big old house with open fires downstairs, the toilets were outside

Table 3 Biographical summaries (Norfolk)

Name	Year Born	School/Training Centre	Hospital	Hostel	Group Home/Flat
Jean Andrews	1942	Village School 1954: Sidestrand	1955: Little Plumstead Hales	1968: Eaton Grange, domestic and factory work	1975: Home 1980: flat, married 2005: Voluntary work
Hilda Peel	1932	Public Assistance Institution	1945: Little Plumstead 1961: Hales	1969: Eaton Grange, domestic work	1974: Home 1990: Private Home 2005: living with a family
Jackie Swinger	1947	1955: Children's Home	1959: Little Plumstead	1968: Eaton Grange, factory work	1970: Lodgings, Group Home Flat: married factory work

Name					
John Andrews	1948	1950: Children's Home	1964: Little Plumstead	1968: Eaton Grange, factory work	1976: Home 1980: Flat married voluntary work
Victor Hall	1932	Public Assistance Institution	1936: Little Plumstead Hall farm work	1956: Blofield daily café and hotel jobs	1972: hotel job 1973: flat 1972: fish and chip shop
Douglas Lanham	1953	Village School Sidestrand School 1957–1969: JTC Great Yarmouth	1971: Blofield Hall 1974: Eaton Grange	1975: hotel job 1980: home 1990: private residential home

and just running with water all the while ... And there didn't seem to be anything done – they all just sat there, I mean it was just somewhere for them to sit. (Rolph, 2002, p. 20)

This seems no improvement over Centres in the 1930s and 1940s. This was not universal, however. Stella Gill eventually enrolled her daughter in the newly opened JTC in Attleborough, South Norfolk, where a combination of close liaison with Special School and a lively parents' group ensured a high standard (Rolph, 2005a). Partly because of the patchy community provision, all six people moved into Little Plumstead Hospital between the 1930s and the 1960s.

Residential services for adults: living arrangements

Jean, Hilda and Jackie all went into Little Plumstead in their early teens, between 1945 and 1959 either because their home life had broken down, or because their families were considered unsuitable to act in a supervisory role. Their lives began to change again before the 1971 White Paper, as a new impetus towards community care encouraged renewed use of Eaton Grange as a way of encouraging young women to move from institution to community. In 1968 and 1969 (a little earlier than Mabel, Gloria and Doris in Croydon) all three moved into Eaton Grange which offered a route – though sometimes a very slow one – towards independent living. The Matron-Manager said:

> Before 1970, Eaton Grange was just seen as ... that was where they would live and that's where they would stay. But everything changed. The aim was, they came in and you tried to teach them how to look after themselves and be in the world and move on and out. (Rolph, 2000, p. 170)

The women revelled in being 'out in the world'. Jackie Swinger remembered: 'When I went to Eaton Grange, I didn't know I was going out into the world. We went into the city ... you just told the staff you were going out ... I got more freedom' (Rolph 2000, p. 173). Jean recalled 'its doors were open! ... I could go out when I liked ... just felt like freedom' (Jean, 2002, p. 207).

After 1971 normalisation (see Chapter 2) encouraged more individuality, although tensions between care and control grew. Jean said that 'towards the end, I felt I was closed in, and wanting to get out, right out. I had more or less freedom in Eaton Grange, but not the freedom I'm getting now here [in her own flat]'(Andrews, 2000). Similarly, regarding

Blofield Hall, some described freedom, while others such as Victor found it oppressive and limiting:

> Moving out ... was a very big change for me. It was a new kind of life ... I was pleased about moving there because we could go out more – we had more freedom than in Plumstead. (Hall and Rolph, 2005, p. 165)

However, Victor resented the control associated with going out:

> we had to write our names down ... We had to be back before 8 o'clock because we used to have roll call, and if we weren't back in time ... we couldn't go into Norwich again ... they locked the doors'. (Hall and Rolph, 2005, p. 168)

Throughout the 1970s, Blofield Hall provided programmes for independence alongside 'an alternative home-life' (Atkinson, 1988). This dual role corresponded to the White Paper's definition of a hostel as a 'permanent home' (Donges, 1982).

The 1971 White Paper, along with the growing critiques of institutions slowly began to influence local policy. But there were few places to move into from the hostels. Private landladies began to fill the gap. Jackie Swinger describes her experience:

> I went to live in W Street with a landlady and two other women from Eaton Grange. I had my own room, but had to pay 5p for a bath or shower. I got my own grub. I gave my money to the landlady to save for me. Then she took the money for her daughter's abortion.[11]

Norfolk Area Health Authority's Strategic Plan (1978) and Joint Working Group Report (1979) described plans for group homes. The 1980s saw the development of 11 group homes; two Social Services hostels; nine private and voluntary homes; and four new ATCs. The increase in availability, combined with successful job placements, meant all six began to move out of hostels. Some Eaton Grange women, including Jackie Swinger, were able to move into flats, thus escaping private landladies. Jackie then married and moved into a council flat where she has lived ever since. Jean Andrews recalled her own final moves:

> I went into a Group Home in about 1975. I was allowed to leave the hostel because I got on, didn't I? And then John [Jean's husband] also came to the Group Home and we stayed for a while until we got this

flat. I worked myself up to get this ... I helped myself. I'd rather have my own place. I couldn't believe my eyes when I saw this flat ... I mean I'd been in those places all that while. And we got married! ... At first when we moved into the flat we had a warden ... I thought we were going to be completely on our own. I put up the flags when they went! We're quite capable of looking after ourselves. (Jean, 2002, pp. 207–8)

These moves would not have been possible unless matched with work and occupation.

Work: daytime occupation

Eaton Grange was described as 'a working hostel'. Domestic work was found for women in the neighbouring houses. Changes took place from the late 1960s. One result of normalisation was the prioritising of ordinary full-time jobs. The route was clear: 'They started by cleaning the church. They liked that and we used to use that as the starting point; then domestic work; then Mackintosh's' (Rolph, 2000, p. 213). In the 1970s, many women worked in Mackintosh's factory, as domestic jobs were phased out. Jean had a full-time job there. She appreciated the increased pay and regular hours. She also understood the crucial role work played in speeding her discharge from the hostel:

> Working was important because it helped us to get out ... for good. Doing a job, helping ourselves, not doing anything wrong ... They said if I helped ... it would probably get me out, which it did, or I wouldn't be here now ...'. (Andrews, 2000, p. 37)

Jackie Swinger worked at the factory until it closed in 1997, but Jean had mixed memories of Mackintosh's:

> There were some bad times and some good times ... But you have to go through it. It was good having a full-time job ... I hated it at Mackintosh's, really hated it, you know. There was a charge hand there and she got onto me ... She said I didn't clean properly ... I used to go into the Tank Room and cry. (Andrews, 2000, p. 39)

Chocolate, clothing, sprout, tin, cracker and shoe factories, and restaurants employed the women and these were the means for them to leave the hostel and move into lodgings, group homes or flats. Work represented a route to an ordinary life.

There was a similar pattern in Blofield Hall. Many men worked on neighbouring farms, but by the early 1970s, Victor, Douglas and John got jobs in Norwich and other nearby towns, as hotel porters, kitchen workers, cleaners in cafes and labourers in boatyards. Factory work remained an option. John Andrews described his first outside job at the cracker factory:

> someone picked us up from Blofield Hall and took us there ... and you had to make the boxes up for the Christmas hampers ... roughly about 4,000 a day! And my hands were aching! And there was a belt. And we put everything in the warehouse onto the belt and the people next door packed them ... and sometimes I used to pack them too. I did get paid for that. We made up the hampers and then we got one free ... I used to like that. (Rolph, 2000, p. 284)

Many men used work to move out of the hostel into live-in work situations and greater independence (Rolph, 2000). A progression route evolved:

> If they wanted to get out badly enough they got to Blofield Hall. The role of the hostels was to get them out, to get them working and to get them out ... They had to earn their way ... they had to climb to the top and the top was the hostel. (Rolph, 2000, p. 290)

The residents saw work as a means to an ordinary life. Douglas Lanham described work as 'a magic wand' and said that 'if you didn't work, you never got out'.

Summary

Community care made slow progress in Norfolk. The two hostels retained a major role, as conduits between hospital and community, as long-term homes for some and half-way houses for others. The six people featured here, having experienced the whole gamut of care, feel that their lives are better now, with more freedom, sometimes better support, and greater opportunities (Jean, 2002; Hall and Rolph, 2005). Hilda has retired, but her new life with a family offers interest and time to enjoy social events. Jean has returned to work as a volunteer in an Oxfam shop. She speaks highly of the support offered by a 'home help' who helps her with household affairs and bills and to prepare for her annual holiday with local friends she has made locally. Victor, now retired, lives in a council flat, attends adult education classes and is involved with self-advocacy. John became involved in voluntary work, and Douglas has retired and lives in a group home close to Jean and Victor.

Conclusion

This chapter has not only demonstrated differences between Croydon and Norfolk but also what they had in common. Community care was implemented in a gradual and piecemeal fashion. Institutional care featured in most of the testimonies. St Lawrence's and Little Plumstead were both linked with their respective hostels and were instrumental in resettling people in their local communities. 'Progression routes' were instituted, taking people from hospital to the community and, where possible, into paid jobs. The recent development of advocacy has seen a further shift – from community care recipient to community participant or citizen.

Notes

1. Norfolk Record Office, Norwich (hereafter NRO): Mental Deficiency Committee minutes (MDCm), 7 May 1946.
2. NRO: Mental Health Services Sub-Committee minutes.
3. Norwich Health Committee, *Annual Report of the MOH, 1963* (Norwich, 1964).
4. 'Lord Mayor's Speech', *Eastern Daily Press*, 24 September 1930.
5. Board of Control Reports, 1923, 1925.
6. NRO: c/mh 1/32 1948.
7. Norwich Health Committee, *Annual Report of the MOH, 1951* (Norwich, 1952).
8. Norwich Health Committee, *Annual Report of the MOH, 1952* (Norwich, 1953).
9. NRO: c/mh 1/35 1951.
10. NRO: Norfolk and Norwich Mencap Society diary, 1977.
11. Interview with Sheena Rolph, 1996.

14
The Voluntary Sector
Liz Tilley

Introduction

This chapter explores the role played by the English voluntary sector in the shaping of community care. It builds on arguments in Chapter 1, that the growth of pressure groups (initially those founded by parents) was both a key driver and a symptom of postwar ideological change. The heterogeneous nature of this sector has permitted it to move freely between the three ideological frameworks of control, care and citizenship. The multiple stakeholders that have constituted the 'voluntary sector' have resulted in highly fluid relationships with the state, as well as fragmentation amongst competing interest groups. Its story has been primarily of a grassroots movement. Both carers and service users have raised their political stake in the development of community-based services through membership of voluntary organisations, particularly since 1971. The sector has provided a means through which their voices have been heard and acknowledged.

From the late 1970s, advocacy became a powerful symbolic player. Advocacy provided a conceptual hook upon which voluntary organisations were able to re-orientate the debate firmly towards the citizenship agenda. It gave rise to what is now being described as the learning disability 'user movement', a range of self-advocacy and user-led groups which have worked to reframe perceptions of the role and value of people with learning disabilities. Their input was a feature of the development of *Valuing People* and remains – at least rhetorically – a significant national directive (DOH, 2001a). However, the extent to which such participation has led self-advocacy organisations to become key players in the strategic planning of services through commissioning, and in service implementation, through service evaluations by users and through Partnership Boards is questionable (Simons, 1999; Clement, 2004).

Despite variance and disunity, a historical analysis of the voluntary sector demonstrates a unique contribution to policy, practice and attitudes. Such organisations are not only agents for change, they are themselves engaged in a process of responding and adapting to wider societal changes (Crossley, 1998). Human geographers in recent years have highlighted 'the strategic importance of space, place and politics for understanding the development and implications of voluntary activity' (Fyfe and Milligan, 2003, p. 398). The chapter alerts readers to the impact that spatial differences may have and acknowledges that we only have a partial view. This is due to the fragmented nature of the sector, which is characterised by a complex – and often area specific – patchwork of groups. This chapter has benefited from the author's research into advocacy organisations in Buckinghamshire. The research demonstrated that the shape of the local voluntary sector was a result of area specific factors, reinforcing this chapter's theme of fragmentation. To gain a more comprehensive picture, additional locally focused research is required.

Insiders and outsiders

Studies of voluntary organisations have adopted a variety of analytical tools including historical (Prochaska, 1988; Lewis, 1995a); economic (Weisbrod, 1988); political (Hadley and Hatch, 1981; Taylor and Lansley, 1992); geographical (Fyfe and Milligan, 2003); and sociological (Saxon-Harrold and Kendall, 1993; Tonkiss and Passey, 1999). Many are generic in their attempts to 'map' the sector (Kendal and Knapp, 1996), but others have addressed the voluntary sector's role within health and social care (Billis and Glennerster, 1998). Crossley's (1998) study of the NAMH in postwar Britain shows it as a 'social movement organisation' which practises 'symbolic violence', a concept developed by Bourdieu (1977) in which organisations attempt to 'impose their discourse or symbolic system upon others, without discussion and in such a way that this discourse becomes accepted as legitimate' (Crossley, 1998, p. 464). Crossley's approach can be employed to explore the impact of wider societal structures on both facilitating and inhibiting the changes sought by other types of voluntary organisations.

Interest in the nature of organisations which occupy a unique position between the public and the private spheres has recently begun to permeate learning disability. The story of the CAMW (a precursor organisation to NAMH) following the 1913 Mental Deficiency Act has been told in terms of its mutually dependent relationship with the statutory authorities (Rooff, 1957; Thomson, 1998a) and its role in the implementation of community-based provision (Walmsley and Rolph, 2001). In a study of the period 1913–59, Walmsley argues that the founding of the NAPBC (termed Mencap henceforth) in 1948 by *parents* of people with learning disabilities marked a watershed, giving rise to a major new group of new stakeholders: the families of people with learning disabilities (Walmsley, 2000a).

Beginnings of a grassroots movement

The expansion of Mencap represented a turning point in the development of community care. It became a powerful campaigning organisation and innovative service provider. It shifted the focus of community care provision away from 'control' and repositioned it within a caring rhetoric. Its success depended on re-imaging people from objects of fear to objects of pity, symbolised by the evocative Little Stephen logo and high-profile advertising campaigns (see Tilley, 1998, 2006).

However, the parents' movement was not confined to Mencap alone. Like Mencap, the National Autistic Society (founded 1962) and the Down Syndrome Association (founded 1970) were largely peopled by 'insiders' (people with a learning disability and their families). Nor has the movement been confined to carers. In 1984, People First London Boroughs was founded, and numerous other user-led groups followed. Mencap paved the way for recognition of the 'insider' voice, and it can be argued that it has engaged in 'symbolic violence' more effectively than any other. But the 'insider voice' has itself become a site of contestation and debate (Tilley, 2006).

The growth of advocacy

The advent of advocacy offered an alternative form of voluntarism. Whilst it has been argued that parents were advocating on behalf of their children long before the term 'advocacy' was coined (Mittler, 1996; Walmsley, 2002, p. 25), 'advocacy' as an activity with a set of prescribed actions and values emerged towards the end of the 1960s in the United States (Flynn and Ward, 1991). Advocacy took hold in the UK a few years later and resulted in the founding of hundreds of schemes encompassing a variety of activities (Atkinson, 1999).

The growth of advocacy broke with earlier developments. Empirical data suggest that schemes have tended to be established by people with an interest in learning disability issues, rather than insiders who have directly experienced them (Wertheimer, 1998; Tilley, forthcoming). There has been an emphasis – articulated first by Wolfensberger and O'Brien, and later adopted by the majority of UK-based advocacy schemes – on encouraging 'valued citizens' and 'ordinary people' to take on the role of advocate (Wolfensberger, 1973; O'Brien, 1982). The renewed importance attributed to the 'active community' in recent years (Griffiths Report, 1988; HMT, 2002) in many ways reflects a key argument of the advocacy movement that such schemes are a two-way process in which significant community development may be realised. In such a model, both the 'volunteer' and the 'recipient' benefit – an interesting evocation of the arguments posited by leading charitable figures and organisations keen to enlist voluntary workers in the inter-war years (Thomson, 1998a, p. 171).

Advocacy has developed within a framework that is notably different to the characteristics that embodied the pre- and interwar CAMW, another 'outsider' voluntary organisation. Walmsley commented: 'members of the CAMW acted largely as an extension of the state's machinery and subjected the private world of the family with a person with a learning disability to public gaze' (Walmsley, 2000a, p. 104). It was at the local level that the close ties between the CAMW and the state were most closely felt. In 1925, there were 351 cases of 'supervision' reported in Buckinghamshire (the monitoring of 'defectives' within the community); 930 in Somerset and only 17 in Bedfordshire, a difference, Walmsley argues, largely attributable to the relative size and zeal of the local branch of the CAMW. Thus CAMW activity levels had an impact on the numbers of individuals and families brought under the care and control of the state in different localities (Walmsley, 2000a).

In contrast, a stipulation for 'pure' citizen advocacy has always been independence from state structures. This remains a highly valued facet of many different types of advocacy, despite being notoriously difficult to achieve. Perhaps more significantly, advocates see their role as promoting citizenship and empowerment, rather than care and protection: 'advocacy is generally acknowledged to play an important, perhaps crucial role in the implementation of community care' (Henderson and Pochin, 2001, p. v). The notion of control that underpinned much of the CAMW's work is alien to advocacy. Nevertheless, there remains a certain degree of fluidity between care, control and citizenship, and the criticism that some advocacy partnerships discourage, rather than promote, empowerment has been made:

> I think you'll find now that the pure citizen advocacy model, as designed and developed by Wolfensberger and O'Brien, there are very

few of those projects still around ... there is some concern about the pure model developing another level of dependency.[1]

I think there's an awful lot of advocacy that still is actually befriending; it's somebody else talking up about what they think is good for the person, rather than truly representing what the person's views are.[2]

Citizen advocacy gained currency due to the weight thrown behind it by journalists and academics in the 1970s and 1980s, such as Ann Shearer and Paul Williams. The movement achieved greater momentum following the uncovering of abuse in learning disability hospitals (Donges, 1982). Later, the concept was forced to mutate and adapt to service users, who began identifying themselves as 'self-advocates'. The early years of the 'official' self-advocacy story have been well documented (Williams and Shoultz, 1982; Hersov, 1996; Goodley, 2000) and indicate that its origins lie in the coming together of a range of stakeholders – including service users, carers and non-disabled support workers. For example, one of the first self-advocacy groups, the Participation Forum set up in 1981, was a Mencap initiative. In the following years a dedicated band of people who came together at the First International Self-Advocacy Conference held in Tacoma, in 1984, visited day and residential services 'teaching' self-advocacy. Self advocates such as Gary Bourlet, along with advisors like John Hersov and Andrea Whittaker, took the concept around the country and encouraged others to start up their own organisations (Hersov, 1996, p. 132).

A number of early initiatives that were not based around specific services were supported by the CMH, now Values into Action, who initially saw the participation of people with learning disabilities as the responsibility of service providers. However, by the mid-1980s this organisation was actively encouraging people to set up their own self-advocacy groups (Barnes, 1997, p. 56). The early years of self-advocacy are characterised by a successful process of reciprocal facilitation and learning. The desire to promote citizenship – a philosophy that having a valued place in the community is a *human right* – has been a powerful link for people who come to these organisations from a range of backgrounds.

State relations

Throughout the twentieth century, different stakeholders in the voluntary sector have gained visibility and power. After 1948, the most prominent constituents were parents. The last two decades of the twentieth century saw some alterations, in part through the growth of different types of advocacy. Voluntary groups that identify themselves as being user-led have developed a much higher profile. This is due both to their success in developing strategies that enable meaningful participation and to a change in Government policy in the 1990s. It has been argued that Government's emphasis on the need to consult the 'consumers' of services has contributed to the emergence of a wider 'user movement' (Barnes et al., 1999). Learning disability user groups reflect the experiences of other organisations such as the disabled people's movement, 'survivors' of mental health services and health consumer groups – many of whom have become increasingly authoritative in their demands (Barnes et al., 1999; Davis, 1999; Baggott et al., 2004). The fluctuating influence of different actors in the learning disability voluntary sector points to a process of continuous renegotiation of the relationship between voluntary associations and statutory bodies, vividly conceptualised by Finlayson (1990) as 'a moving frontier'.

Since the late 1980s, historians of British social policy have reassessed the dominant historical narrative of previous years which presented the 'classic welfare state' era as the triumph of collectivism over individualism and of statutory rights over philanthropic benevolence. A review of the voluntary sector's role in the mixed provision of welfare has indicated that the postwar 'consensus' years may have been something of an anomaly (Digby, 1989; Lowe, 2005). Lewis has argued that 'the pattern of voluntary and statutory activity was unpredictable' in the prewar years and by no means demonstrates a clear division in which voluntary organisations had the dominant role in providing social care (Lewis, 1995b, p. 15). This position is borne out in Thomson's work on 'the problem of mental deficiency', in which he explains the 'symbiotic' relationship between the CAMW and Board of Control (Thomson, 1998a). The Mental Deficiency Act certainly redistributed – if not intentionally curbed – voluntary influence, as the sector ceded control of institutions in return for a 'quasi-official remit' for community care after 1913 (Walmsley, 2000a, p. 108).

An appraisal of the literature on state-voluntary relationships after 1948 suggests that this was a period in which the state became the dominant player in the provision of welfare services (Brenton, 1985). Although the Wolfenden Report of 1978 recommended an expanded role for the voluntary sector, it has been pointed out that for reasons ranging from pragmatism to ideology, Social Services Departments were often reluctant to yield a greater stake to voluntary organisations in the provision of such services (Lewis, 1995a). However, whilst local authorities in theory maintained a monopoly over community care services for people with learning disabilities before 1971, prior to that date local groups innovated alternative forms of community care and developed working partnerships with statutory bodies in order to fund and manage their services (see below). These organisations have carved a distinct niche for themselves, sometimes wholly separate from state structures, but frequently in partnership with them. The increase in project funding, first through the grant system, and later through contractual specification and tendering of 'services', has created another dynamic in the statutory-voluntary relationship, which has created as many difficulties as it has opportunities for voluntary organisations.

Campaigning

Crucial to the story of postwar voluntary organisations for people with learning disabilities has been campaigning. Mencap began as a campaigning organisation, lobbying for the introduction of mandatory education for children (Shennan, 1980, p. 10). It demanded help for mothers caring for their children at home, as well as more day services and Occupation Centres, arguing that care in the community could only work if support systems were in place for families. It was called to give evidence in 1954 to the Royal Commission, a first in terms of national policy influence. Mencap was creating an organisational profile in these early years that was built upon its ability to challenge the assumed knowledge of those in authority. It developed international networks, which allowed it to channel advances in community care provision from areas such as Scandinavia and the US back into the UK. In 1969, Bank-Mikkelsen of the Danish National Mental Retardation Service was invited to speak at its annual general meeting (*Parents Voice*, December 1969, p. 17). The following year, in a press release, George Lee, General-Secretary of the NSMHCA, commented:

> Despite all our advances over the last few years in day care provision for the Mentally Handicapped ... there is no gainsaying the fact that, in the matter of residential care, we are being hopelessly outpaced by the more advanced countries of Europe, such as Sweden and Denmark. (*Parents Voice*, December 1970, p. 8)

The 1971 White Paper credited the NSMHCA as being a prominent organisation responsible for changing attitudes towards people with learning disabilities, and it was invited to make comments on the document in draft stage (Donges, 1982, p. 121). Mencap continued to campaign on a range of issues, from improved residential provision to respite care; the continued refinement of education services for children with learning disabilities and, in the 1980s, the legal right for people to have an independent advocate. It also put up a ferocious battle against cuts to Social Services Departments in the late 1970s and early 1980s.

Other organisations have subsequently taken up the campaigning mantle and adopted more radical and challenging positions. Self-advocacy groups have lobbied both central and local government on policies including independent living, Direct Payments and accessible information. In 1986, following a consultation with People First, a 'simple English' version of the Disabled Persons Representation Bill was produced (Hersov, 1996, p. 134). Such actions have established user organisations as political agents, which have helped shift the ideological framework of community care towards one which values people's rights to have a stake in decisions which affect their everyday life. As Barnes (1997, p. 58) commented, the push towards Direct Payments infused the community care debate with an 'explicit consumerist philosophy', which resonated powerfully with other user interest groups. However, Crossley highlights the difficulties of ascertaining the causes of policy initiatives (Crossley, 1998). The degree to which voluntary organisations have impacted upon policy developments in learning disability – both before and after 1971 – is not clear because they are but one of many stakeholders. However, as Chapter 1 indicates, it certainly played a significant role in stimulating changes in the ideological climate.

Service provision

From the 1950s onwards, Mencap branches were involved in running services, ranging from welfare visitors to social clubs (Rolph, 2002). Some went further and invested in the development of residential homes and Training Centres, managed either by local branch members, or by local authority employees. The Norwich and District Mencap Society set up two Industrial Centres, one for men and one for women, which were eventually taken over by the local authority (Rolph, 2005c). Partnerships between local Mencap groups and local authorities became common practice, with the organisation raising funds to develop pioneering schemes, on the understanding that the local authority would finance their continued maintenance. These service blueprints were undoubtedly innovative, but were overwhelmingly inspired by a 'caring' discourse. A pamphlet in national Mencap's archives describing the early years of its well-known sheltered hostel and Training Centre in

Slough explains that the centre consisted of two villas, each for a 'family of severely handicapped young men and women, between the ages of 16 and 26', which would have a set of 'house-parents' to oversee them. It goes on:

> Here, by the careful integration of work and social training, and by the expert encouragement of 'parents', trainees proceed in a practical situation as a group towards social competence. (NSMHCA pamphlet, nd)

The Slough project gained national attention for its demonstration that people with learning disabilities were able to undertake work activities in community-based settings. However, the language is laden with paternalistic overtones and implies a reluctance to regard people as capable adults.

In the Silver Jubilee edition of *Parents Voice* in 1971, the National Chairman of the NSMHCA, Lord Segal, commented:

> Today we are still painfully aware of how much more remains to be done. We can, however, face the future with some degree of confidence. Let us now redouble our efforts to achieve even greater progress in the years to come. (*Parents Voice*, December, 1971, p. 5)

At the beginning of the 1970s, the unsatisfactory nature of community care services, combined with the institutional scandals and sociological research that emerged at the end of the previous decade (Morris, 1969; *Report of the Committee of Inquiry*, 1969) forced Mencap to reflect upon its role as a lobby group, as well as the extent of its success in seeking to influence Government policy. Over the next ten years it made increasingly detailed and ambitious plans for direct service provision, which culminated in the launch of the Homes Foundation project at the beginning of the 1980s (*Parents Voice*, Winter 1980–81, p. 4).

The decision to extend the provision of services for people with learning disabilities, improve quality and offer services where the state was not active corresponds with broader developments occurring within the voluntary sector at this time (outlined above). However, some facets of Mencap's changing role became contentious. There were a number of administrative difficulties, many of which have been the cause of underlying tensions between national Mencap and its local branches (*Parents Voice*, 1987).[3] This reorientation towards an expanded care provider role instigated a new organisational phase for Mencap – one in which it became open to challenge on the quality of its own provision.

Advocacy schemes were designed to provide a mechanism through which people could become valued members of the community, rather than merely existing on its fringes in the 'eternal child' role (Wolfensberger, 1972). Although advocacy has been integral to the development of community-based services since the late 1970s, it has not been recognised as a statutory right for people with learning disabilities (Atkinson, 1999, p. 41). Despite the importance attributed to independence in advocacy literature, in reality most advocacy organisations rely in part, if not wholly, on funds from local and national government. Whilst *Valuing People* ring-fenced money specifically for advocacy schemes, applications exceeded resources, resulting in the continued tie of many organisations to their local Health Authorities and Social Services Departments, often with the associated conflict of interests:

> The majority of our funding does come from service providers ... On one occasion we were told that our funding would be under threat if we continued to use one of the advocates. But we did, and they didn't cut the funding. Or perhaps over the years they have down-marked us ... So, that's one of the reasons I feel uneasy about the fact our main funding comes from there – but it's difficult to find it anywhere else.[4]

Initially advocacy schemes were financed through grants. However, the onset of the contract culture during the 1990s led to the increasing use of Service Level Agreements and tendering processes for advocacy 'services'. The introduction of Best Value in April 2000 heightened the need for contractual specifications in an environment in which statutory funders must demonstrate evidence of 'economy, efficiency and effectiveness' (DETR, 1999, p. 3; Henderson and Pochin, 2001). In 1992, following the introduction of the purchaser/provider split, a Social Services Department, which was recognised as being a front runner in restructuring the way it financed voluntary organisations, commented that there would be some activities for which grants would always be more appropriate. These included the work of advocacy and self-help groups, for whom outcomes were hard to measure (Edwards, 1992, p. 29). But now most advocacy services are contractual.

This funding scenario poses difficulties for advocacy groups on two fronts. Organisations frequently become dependent on statutory funding streams, meaning a loss of independence, and the 'conditions' attached to such funds creates further problems. Emphasis on performance indicators, unit costs and deliverable outputs encourage a climate of accountability which seem to be accepted by voluntary groups, but these conditions also threaten the sense of independence, control and creativity that are an essential part of their organisational identity. As Fyfe and Milligan argue, 'the increasing dependence of voluntary organisations on state grants and contracts, combined with increased administrative oversight and regulatory control, may simply reinforce state authority over welfare provision and may lead to an increase in state penetration of everyday activities' (Fyfe and Milligan, 2003, p. 401). In these circumstances, advocacy organisations find themselves in the paradoxical situation of developing an agenda of 'choice and independence' which has been conceptualised from the statutory perspective.

Fragmentation

A significant aspect of the voluntary sector for people with learning disabilities has been diversity. Prior to the Second World War, the CAMW had something of a monopoly. Since then a huge variety of organisations has emerged. Some have an established a national profile, while many remain powerful at the local level. Within this spectrum, tensions have surfaced, and disunity has frequently been around issues of representation. Some parents have moved away from generic organisations such as Mencap and have founded groups which address the specific health and social care needs of their children. The advocacy movement has historically been beset with divisions around 'pure' and 'practical' advocacy, as well as conflicts between the respective advantages and disadvantages of expressive and instrumental approaches. As Henderson and Pochin have pointed out, this means that after 25 years there are no national advocacy standards available, and the movement lacks a clear identity (Henderson and Pochin, 2001, p. 14).

> There have been lots of squabbles around advocacy ... And also because you've got a fundamental argument that regardless of whether it's self-advocacy or advocacy, if you're setting up an organisation based on user empowerment, then users should have control. And the advocacy organisations have been run by people who run advocacy organisations, rather than users. And then you get to the situation of well, which users?[5]

Carers have criticised user-led organisations for focusing only on the 'most-able' service users, leading to the reproduction of a 'hierarchy of disability' that has also pervaded the physical disability movement (Deal, 2003).

> I think one of the greatest fears of parents ... is that self-advocacy is only for those people who can communicate very easily, you know – the most able. And that people with higher support needs couldn't possibly speak for themselves and make choices, and that it would have to be their parents that made those choices.[6]

For a number of parents, there has been anxiety around the perception that advocacy organisations overrule a parent's involvement in their child's life:

> Well, I sat with S, while the parents that were there accused me of briefing her to say that she wanted to be involved in this consulta- tion, and it was obvious that she couldn't get involved, and none of them could get involved, and what could they say, and why was I pushing this? I got abusive telephone calls at home and all sorts of things. And that was trying to get people with learning difficulties involved.[7]

Likewise, the user movement has challenged other voluntary organisa- tions over their entitlement to speak on behalf of service users, and has criticised the representation of people with learning disabilities by some of the parent-founded groups (Shearer, 1986, p. 181). Self-advocacy's underlying principle of empowering people with learning disabilities to achieve adult status means that the potential for conflict with parent groups is high (Barnes, 1997, p. 55). However, there is some evidence of the dilution of such tensions:

> Something happened recently, with one of the carers who'd been previously a bit difficult – this guy was part of the group of carers that had been a bit suspicious of us in the past. But we found out recently that he'd been going round doing a lot of work with the older carers on self-advocacy. So yes, relationships have improved with carers.[8]

> People [service users] have been their own ambassadors, there's no doubt about it, and they've changed lots of people's views. And they've created an environment where they state very clearly 'there's room for everybody here'. Yes, carers are really, really important, and they must have a voice, but it mustn't be to the exclusion of people with learning disabilities. And now we do have a much better work- ing relationship with carers' groups than we did have.[9]

Nevertheless, the question of which user-led groups are most 'representative' remains contentious:

> You will have a self-advocacy group at the Partnership Board, and they're sent to the Partnership Board to represent all people with a learning disability. And sometimes you think, right, hold on a minute, you're speaking up for yourself, but you also represent people with a learning disability – what advocacy is that?[10]

Has this disunity been damaging? Within the context of advocacy, arguments have been made that disunity has resulted in a worrying lack of consistency and coherence, which threatens its ability to influence policy and practice (Henderson and Pochin, 2001, p. 14). However, tensions have also infused advocacy with dynamism which has aided its expansion. User-led groups have failed, after a number of attempts, to create a national organisation for England. Many are concerned primarily with issues of a local significance and have not been persuaded of the potential benefits of joining forces. Whilst this may provide evidence of the movement's inability to reconcile its differences, it also points to the strong identity of these local groups, which have developed defined roles and structures to influence the services that have a direct impact on them.

Conclusion

This chapter has explored the role played by the voluntary sector in the development of community care for people with learning disabilities since 1948. It has demonstrated its complexity, and the difficulties of mapping its changing constituents and their contributions. Different groups have challenged the assumptions of community care policy at various historical points, oscillating between the three ideological frameworks of control, care and citizenship and have played an important role in shaping its implementation. The relationship with the state has been fluid. These organisations have both responded to and influenced the community care agenda. The chapter has highlighted the difficulties of assessing the sector's impact on policy developments. There have been a range of actors, institutions and wider structural forces beyond the voluntary sector pushing change. Most voluntary organisations share the aim of improving the lives of people with learning disabilities. Yet ideas about how this might be achieved have varied enormously between groups, leading to internal dissent. And yet these different organisations continue to thrive and develop ideas in a period of financial insecurity, in which more organisations than ever before are competing for limited funds. Historically, these organisations have criticised and challenged one other. Despite, or perhaps because of this, the voluntary sector has become a powerful and multi-vocal presence, which has undoubtedly contributed to the changing face of community care in British social policy.

Notes

1. Interview in 2005 with the Project Manager of People's Voices – a Buckinghamshire-based advocacy organisation.
2. Interview in 2005 with the *Valuing People* Strategy Manager, Buckinghamshire County Council.
3. Oral history interview with Joan Levingson, Barnet Mencap, 2000.
4. Interview in 2005 with the Project Manager of People's Voices.
5. Ibid.
6. Interview in 2004 with the Chief Executive of Talkback.
7. Interview in 2005 with the Project Manager of People's Voices.
8. Interview in 2005 with the Project Coordinator of Talkback.
9. Interview in 2004 with the Chief Executive of Talkback.
10. Interview in 2005 with the Executive Manager of the Integrated Learning Disability Services, Buckinghamshire County Council.

Conclusion

John Welshman and Jan Walmsley

Introduction

This book has set out to tell the story of how, in the relatively short period of 50 years, 1948–2001, the fortunes of people with learning difficulties changed quite dramatically. It has primarily been a story of what happened in the United Kingdom, although Part III of the book has also addressed developments in other parts of the Western world, highlighting significant convergences. The book has examined community care, the growth of services, through the lenses provided by our core themes of care, control and citizenship. Furthermore we have tried to look beneath the surface by focusing not just on policy but at the experiences of people with learning difficulties and those of their families. Here, in the Conclusion, we draw together the threads of the book and reflect upon the relevance of the book to contemporary care. We try to sum up some of our arguments by focusing on four themes: the forces for change; the core themes of care, control and citizenship; comparing community care for people with learning difficulties with other types of service users; and finally, the practice of social history itself.

The forces for change

In explaining the emergence of care in the community as a policy option in this period, it is important to recognise that its origins lie in the interwar period, or earlier. Much care was, and has continued to be, provided by the family. However we have also seen various forces for change operating in our period. First, rarely recognised in the 'official' story, but an important part of our distinctive approach, were the efforts of the families themselves, usually parents campaigning for improved services for their children, articulated through local voluntary Societies from the early 1950s. Although assessing the exact impact of these organisations on policy development is difficult, there is no doubt that they were an important force, more organised and vocal than they had been in the interwar period. Related to this was the rise to prominence of user groups, notably People First, a late twentieth-century phenomenon which brought issues relating to 'rights' and 'citizenship' to the fore.

Second, we have seen the power of ideas. Before the Second World War, arguably the dominant ideological influence on mental deficiency policy and practice was that of eugenics. Nevertheless in the postwar period there was significant movement in the ideological climate, informed in part by research. The Campaign waged by the NCCL in 1950 exposed exploitation and restriction of the liberty of patients within institutions, evidence of a change in the attitudes of the general public, and based in part on individualistic human rights ideology. Moreover in the period up to 1971, research increasingly discredited the existing system of care, by illustrating the flawed system of classification and highlighting the potential for training and rehabilitation to make a difference; demonstrating the potential of alternative forms of care provision; and demolishing the idea of the institution as a therapeutic environment. This research, chiefly emanating from social psychology, was broadened by sociological critiques of institutional life, notably Goffman's *Asylums* (1961), but augmented in the UK by *Put Away* (1969). Finally the period since 1971 had been heavily influenced by normalisation, effectively feeding into the theme of citizenship as articulated in *Valuing People*.

Third there was the influence of scandals. It is doubtful whether the impetus for change would have been so rapid had it not been for the Ely Hospital, Cardiff, scandal in 1967, and perhaps more importantly the *Report of the Committee of Inquiry* under Geoffrey Howe (1969). It was not so much the impact of the scandal *per se*, though this certainly affected knowledge of such issues on the part of the general public, but the way concern was translated into action at the national policy level. Under Richard Crossman, then Secretary of State for Social Services, the whole report was published, leading directly to the setting up of a Working Party, and in time, to the establishment of the Hospital Advisory Service. Up to that point, progress had been slow, under the *Hospital Plan* and *Health and Welfare* White Papers. Arguably it remained equally slow thereafter, but scandals were an important force on the Ministry of Health, later the DHSS.

Fourth there was the issue of costs. Much of the current secondary literature on the history of care in the community focuses on the history of people with mental health needs (Sedgwick, 1982; Scull, 1984; Busfield, 1986; Unsworth, 1987; Bartlett and Wright, 1999). One of the main areas of debate has been over the relative importance of the economic costs of care, on the one hand, and the development of pharmacology, on the other, as twin forces underpinning the emergence of care in the community as a policy option. There is no doubt that the perceived costs of care in institutions was a feature of policymaking in this period, perhaps most obviously in the late 1950s and early 1960s, when cost-cutting was an attractive option for the Conservative Right. Similar points have been made in Chapters 6 and 7, in the case of the USA, Norway and Sweden. Nevertheless as Sedgwick has argued (1982), the fiscal crisis was arguably more a feature of the 1970s than the 1950s, and again this impacted on policy development for people with learning disabilities.

It is one of the most striking messages of this book that these different pressures to close institutions worked almost simultaneously across the countries highlighted in Part III. The growth of parental pressure groups, scandals and the interest of the press in conditions for inmates of institutions led across the Western world to a movement which discredited, not just 'bad apples' in institutions, but the system and philosophy of care it represented. Faltering steps towards community provision also characterise the countries represented in this book. Shifts from regarding community provision as mere adjuncts to institutions, increasing diversity of providers, the growth of a consumer-oriented, rights-based individualistic approach and individualised packages of care all show remarkable convergence.

Care, control and citizenship

When we started to write the book, we had in our minds a fairly straightforward trajectory which saw services in 1948 being about control, gradually shading into 'care' with the 1971 White Paper, and shifting from then to the end of the century towards a citizenship model. If these themes are helpful as a way of characterising different eras, 'control' seems best to fit the period up to 1948, when as noted above eugenics was arguably the dominant influence on policy and practice. The forms of care in the community that were pioneered following the 1913 Act – guardianship, supervision and licence – were arguably more about protecting society from people with learning difficulties, and to a lesser extent about protecting people with learning difficulties from society, than with 'care' in any meaningful sense. Similarly 'care' would on the face of it appear to capture some of the significant policy initiatives and organisational changes in the period 1948–71, when, whether carried through into practice or not, these had 'better care' as their driving rationale. Finally 'citizenship' appeared to us a way of defining the period since 1971, with significant changes in models of disability and attitudes to 'rights' and 'citizenship' being symbolised by the publication of *Valuing People* at the end of our period.

Nevertheless while tempting to offer this kind of overview, the reality is very different. The three themes may describe national policy intentions reasonably accurately, but as we got into the grain of survivor's accounts, and into in-depth descriptions of services (Jones, 1975; Carter, 1981), we realised that it was a much more nuanced picture. In support of this contention, we would offer three illustrations, that, we would argue, represent important elements of continuity rather than change.

First, there is the theme of staffing at the local level, where there were significant elements of continuity with the pre-NHS era. The MWOs appointed by local authorities in the 1950s were often unqualified former Poor Law ROs. Oral evidence has indicated that they perceived their job as being as much about control as care, with physical strength, for instance, being seen as an important prerequisite. Similarly the wardens of local authority hostels either often had no qualifications or had similar experience of other kinds of institutions. In contrast a qualified workforce in the form of social workers was very slow to develop as some commentators recognised (Titmuss, 1961). Similar continuities characterised the history of learning disability nursing. Indeed there is much evidence that these problems in staffing persisted into our final period, and up to the present day.

Second, we would point to the emphasis on industrial work rather than education and rehabilitation, which it is clear pervaded local authority JTCs and ATCs, and the work performed by the residents of local authority hostels. One of the most prominent aspects of local authority provision was the Occupation Centre of the 1950s. Despite the creation of JTCs in the 1960s, children only came under LEA supervision in 1971. In this respect, there is evidence that the UK lagged behind other European comparator countries, such as the Netherlands, although it was in this respect in step with Canada, the USA and Australia. Despite the contribution of research by social psychologists, which from the 1950s demonstrated that people with learning disabilities could and should perform much more complex tasks, evidence suggests that the nature of work in the ATCs in particular was dictated more by the needs of local industrial firms, through contracts, than by the needs of the services users themselves. Again oral history interviews have suggested that work continued to be seen as a form of atonement rather than as a stepping stone to a 'normal' life (Rolph, 2000).

Third, there is the question of the reality of social interaction for people with learning difficulties themselves. There were continual attempts to create appropriate environments; the 1971 White Paper, for example, urged that the hostel should be more like a home. Nevertheless the extent to which hostels acted as half-way houses between the institution and the community is more open to question. Similarly despite the impact of normalisation and SRV in the 1970s, a survey published in 2005 indicated that despite *Valuing People*, the reality of social interaction for people with learning disabilities themselves was very limited (Emerson *et al.*, 2005). Thus while clearly a more sustained analysis is desirable, we would argue that these three brief illustrations serve to cast considerable doubt on the utility of the themes of care, control and citizenship, indicating significant elements of continuity alongside change. Control could masquerade as care; care often contained important elements of control; and citizenship often was a shifting discourse located somewhere between the twin poles of control and care, more aspirational than actual.

The UK in international perspective

The timeline (pp. xiii–xxi) reveals interesting points of contact between the experience of the UK and other parts of the Western world. The USA appears to follow a similar chronology, with books by parents and others in the 1950s and early 1960s; the slow development of services in the 1960s, inspired by budget cuts and criticisms of conditions in institutions; and legislation in the 1970s. In Canada, too, the 1950s saw experimental schools and the formation of the OARC in 1953. Ontario's institution population peaked in 1964, and the HRP Act and VRA followed in 1966. Similarly the Martel and Sanderson tragedies in 1971 led directly to the Williston Report, and this coincided with Wolf Wolfensberger's visit to the National Institute for Mental Retardation, in Toronto. The Developmental Services Act was passed in 1974 and Bill 82 in 1980. The deadline for the closure of institutions in Ontario is, at the time of writing, 2007.

Norway and Sweden, on the other hand, had seen some legislation in the 1950s, but little until the late 1960s. The number of residents of institutions peaked in Sweden and Denmark in 1970; in Norway, Finland and Iceland in 1976. In the 1980s, there were Public Committee Reports, in

Norway and Sweden, and legislation, and the year 2000 was set for the closure of institutions in Sweden. Judging Australia through the case-study of Victoria, there appeared to be little activity until the Intellectually Disabled Persons Services and Guardianship and Administration Board Acts of 1986. A three-year plan was published in 1989 and an Intellectual Disability Services Task Force established in 1995.

Of course space here has permitted consideration only of the USA, Canada, Norway and Sweden and Australia, and two of these have of necessity been case studies. Nevertheless despite differences in chronology between the different countries, there are also striking points of comparison. These include the importance of the exposés of conditions in institutions, including in newspapers and periodicals (USA, Canada and UK); the impact of publications by parents (USA and UK); the formation of local and national voluntary groups (UK, USA and Canada); the dominance of normalisation (Denmark, Norway, Sweden, UK and Canada); the growth of advocacy movements (USA and UK); and the emergence of alternative forms of provision through legislation and planning documents (all). All of the five countries or regions featured in the book followed a similar trajectory, although at different speeds. What this illustrates is the potential of international comparative studies of the history of care in the community for people with learning difficulties. The aim here has been a modest one, primarily to provide a context for the development of services in the UK, but the comparative potential of this field is clear.

People with learning difficulties, mental health and older people

Much of the current secondary literature on the history of care in the community focuses on the history of people with mental health needs. Other work has focused on the development of services for older people, especially through the expansion of domiciliary services (Means and Smith, 1985). And more recently the theme of disability, particularly physical disability, has been emphasised (Borsay, 2005). By contrast, the experiences of people with learning difficulties have been comparatively neglected.

Separating the experiences of people with learning difficulties from those with mental health needs is difficult, especially in the earlier part of the period when the two were often conflated in both policy documents at the national level and in the organisation of services at the local level. Local authority Mental Health Committees, for example, covered both services for people with learning difficulties and for those with mental health needs. James Trent has shown that people with learning difficulties in the USA benefited from the exposé of conditions in institutions for patients with mental health needs. Similarly leaving aside differences in life expectancy between different social groups, people with mental health needs and those with learning difficulties do ultimately become older people. There are dangers, therefore, in dividing people up into distinctive groups according to their entitlements to specific components of care provision and services.

Nevertheless part of our argument is that the experiences of people with learning difficulties are a distinctive part of the story of care in the community in general. While the perceived economic costs of institutional care undoubtedly were a factor in the move to care in the community, the development of pharmacological forms of care, such as tranquillisers, were of relatively little significance in the case of learning disability. Moreover part of our argument has been that there has been an increasing divergence between services for people with mental health needs and for those with learning difficulties through our period. That is not to say that each has not influenced the other. But certainly the conflation of the two in both policy evolution and service delivery is much less apparent in the period since 1971 than in the preceding years. This appears to be symbolised in the fact that the two groups of service users had their own White Papers by the early 1970s (DHSS, 1971, 1975), a trend that prevailed into the twenty-first century with the warmly welcomed *Valuing People* representing a very different set of values and service imperatives to the controversial and troubled (at the time of writing) proposal to replace the 1983 Mental Health Act in England.

The practice of social history

The book has drawn on the distinctive approach of the Social History of Learning Disability Group at the Open University, mixing autobiographical, oral and life history approaches with more traditional archival and documentary sources to provide a comprehensive account of care in the community. The 'official' story of the history of care in the community in the postwar period is reasonably well known, albeit better in the case of older people and people with mental health needs rather than people with learning difficulties (Means and Smith, 1994; Bartlett and Wright, 1999; Means *et al.*, 2003; Borsay, 2005). In part this reflects the availability of archives for the key Government departments responsible for the main policy initiatives (Bridgen and Lowe, 1998). Nevertheless while there has been a huge volume of work recovering the voice of people with learning disabilities themselves, and to a lesser extent that of the workforce, to date the 'official' and 'user' stories have not been integrated in one narrative. The difference is not so much one of sources, since the work on 'user' accounts has contextualised oral evidence with local archival materials and other published sources (Rolph *et al.*, 2003). Rather it has been of deciding the relative importance of different voices within the dominant narrative.

At one point in the writing of this book we considered starting with the 'Experiences' and then using this to lead on to the sections on 'Ideology and Ideas' and 'Organisations and Structures'. In the end we rejected this, considering it too disorientating for readers. What we have tried to do instead has been to start with the more conventional narratives, using more traditional sources, but to demonstrate the connections between these and the themes taken up more fully in 'Experiences'. In part, we have found that the task of integrating the two narratives has served to throw up new ideas and themes, a process of cross fertilisation that we have found extremely stimulating. Oral history has had a crucial function in the history of learning disability, by filling in details that archives usually fail to deliver, and through by-passing the established record with testimony from eye witness accounts.

Nevertheless we argue that it is important to move the argument about oral history on, from the question of disputed ownership, to issues of reliability and validity. In some respects oral history has been used to bolster preconceptions, rather than challenge them, for example in focusing on the 'good' families rather than those who were abusive, neglectful or uncaring, and by failing to give a voice to those who liked institutional life, and regretted its demise (Rolph and Walmsley, 2006). We argue strongly that the task of uncovering the voice of the service user has largely been completed; a more interesting but more demanding job is to integrate that with the 'official' story. The task now is more to integrate the documentary and oral evidence more effectively, rather than juxtaposing the one against the other, in seeing the oral evidence as in some way superior to the dull archival sources. While recognising that our more radical plans for reordering the book were perhaps premature, we feel that we have gone some way towards that enterprise in this book, particularly through the service users' accounts, including those told through pictures and forms of reminiscence other than the spoken or written, in Part IV.

Conclusion

In the Introduction we said that we were setting out to explore an extraordinary historical transition, between 1948 and 2001, in the fortunes of people with learning difficulties. In 1948, highly negative imagery of people with learning difficulties predominated, and the community care provision that did exist was seen, not as a means of enabling people to be part of society, but as an adjunct to institutional provision. In 2001, on the other hand, *Valuing People* identified independence, choice, rights and inclusion as the proper objectives of policy. Community-based services were the means by which these were to be achieved, and beyond Government policy, aspirations were being expressed for full citizenship. We also said that in looking at experiences as well as policy, we would question whether the surface changes were any more than that. Overall, we would conclude our book by arguing that while there has been an extraordinary historical transition, in terms of the growth of services acting as a means for inclusion and rights, things have not changed so dramatically for people with learning difficulties and their families. It has been more the promise of change, achieved to a remarkable degree for some, but for many, it remains just that – a promise.

References

Abbott, P., and Sapsford, R. (1987), *Community Care for Mentally Handicapped Children*, London: Croom Helm.

Abbs, G. (2005), 'You Have Been a Mother to Him: We Could Only Have Been an Uncle', in Rolph *et al.* (eds), *Witnesses to Change*, pp. 37–9.

Abrams, P. (1977), 'Community Care: Some Research Problems and Priorities', *Policy and Politics*, vol. 6, 125–51.

Adams, M., and Lovejoy, H. (1972), *The Mentally Subnormal: Social Work Approaches* (2nd edn), London: Heinemann Medical Books.

Allsop, J. (1984), *Health Policy and the National Health Service*, Harlow: Longman.

American Association on Mental Retardation (1992), *Mental Retardation: Definition, Classification and Systems of Support* (9th edn), Washington: American Association on Mental Retardation.

Andrews, C. (2005), 'Pay and Dismay', *Community Care*, 26 May, 32–3.

Andrews, J. (1996), 'Identifying and Providing for the Mentally Disabled in Early Modern London', in Digby and Wright (eds), *From Idiocy to Mental Deficiency*, pp. 65–92.

Andrews, J., with Rolph, S. (2000), 'Scrub, Scrub, Scrub ... Bad Times and Good Times: Some of the Jobs I've Had in my Life', in Atkinson *et al.* (eds), *Good Times, Bad Times*, pp. 31–42.

Angell, S. L. Jr (1944), 'Training School – And CPS', *Reporter* III, 15 July, 3–5.

Anglin, B., and Braaten, J. (1978), *Twenty-Five Years of Growing Together: A History of the Ontario Association for the Mentally Retarded*, Toronto: Canadian Association for the Mentally Retarded.

Apte, R. (1968), *Halfway Houses: A New Dilemma in Institutional Care*, London: G. Bell & Sons.

Armitage, A. (1975), *Social Welfare in Canada*, Toronto: McClelland Stewart.

Aspis, S. (2000), 'Researching our History: Who is in Charge?', in Brigham *et al.* (eds), *Crossing Boundaries*, pp. 1–5.

Atkinson, D. (1988), 'Residential Care for Children and Adults with Mental Handicap', in Sinclair (ed.), *The Research Reviewed*, pp. 125–56.

Atkinson, D. (1997), 'Learning from Local History: Evidence from Somerset', in Atkinson *et al.* (eds), *Forgotten Lives*, pp. 107–25.

Atkinson, D. (1998a), 'Autobiography and Learning Disability', *Oral History*, vol. 26, no. 1, 73–80.

Atkinson, D. (1998b), 'Reclaiming Our Past: Empowerment through Oral History and Personal Stories', in Ward (ed.), *Innovations in Advocacy and Empowerment*.

Atkinson, D. (1998c), 'Living in Residential Care', in Brechin, Walmsley, Katz, and Peace (eds), *Care Matters: Concepts, Practice and Research in Health and Social Care*, London: Sage, pp. 13–26.

Atkinson, D. (1999), *Advocacy: A Review*, Brighton: Joseph Rowntree Foundation/ Pavilion.

Atkinson, D. (2002), 'Self-Advocacy and Research', in B. Gray and R. Jackson (eds), *Advocacy and Learning Disability*, London: Jessica Kingsley, pp. 120–36.

Atkinson, D., and Cooper, M. (2000), 'Parallel Stories', in Brigham *et al.* (eds), *Crossing Boundaries*, pp. 15–25.

Atkinson, D., and Walmsley, J. (1999), 'Using Autobiographical Approaches with People with Learning Disabilities', *Disability and Society*, vol. 14, no. 2, 203–17.

Atkinson, D., and Williams, F. (eds) (1990), *Know Me As I Am: An Anthology of Prose, Poetry and Art by People with Learning Difficulties*, London: Hodder and Stoughton.

Atkinson, D., Jackson, M., and Walmsley, J. (eds) (1997), *Forgotten Lives: Exploring the History of Learning Disability*, Kidderminster: BILD Publications.

Atkinson, D., McCarthy, M., Walmsley, J., Cooper, M., Rolph, S., Barette, P., Coventry, M., and Ferris, G. (2000), *Good Times, Bad Times: Women with Learning Difficulties Telling Their Stories*, Kidderminster: BILD Publications.

Audit Commission (1986), *Making a Reality of Community Care*, London: HMSO.

Ayer, S., and Alaszewski, A. (1984), *Community Care for the Mentally Handicapped: Services for Mothers and their Mentally Handicapped Children*, London: Croom Helm.

Baggott, R., Allsop, J., and Jones, K. (2004), 'Representing the Repressed? Health Consumer Groups and the National Policy Process', *Policy and Politics*, vol. 32, no. 3, 317–32.

Bank-Mikkelson, N. E. (1969). 'Modern Service Models', in *Changing Patterns in Residential Services for the Mentally Retarded*, Washington DC: President's Committee on Mental Retardation.

Bank-Mikkelson, N. E. (1980), 'Denmark', in Flynn and Nitsch (eds), *Normalisation, Social Integration and Community Services*, pp. 51–70.

Baranyay, E. P. (1971), *The Mentally Handicapped Adolescent: The Slough Project of the National Society for Mentally Handicapped Children: An Experimental Step Towards Life in the Community*, Oxford: Pergamon Press.

Barnes, M. (1997), *Care, Communities and Citizens*, Harlow: Addison Wesley Longman.

Barnes, M., Harrison, S., Mort, M., and Shardlow, P. (1999), *Unequal Partners: User Groups and Community Care*, Bristol: Policy Press.

Barron, D. (1996), *A Price to be Born*, Harrogate: Mencap, Northern Division.

Bartlett, P., and Wright, D. (eds.) (1999), *Outside the Walls of the Asylum: The History of Care in the Community 1750–2000*, London: Athlone.

Barton, R. (1961), 'The Institutional Mind and the Subnormal Mind', *British Journal of Mental Subnormality*, vol. 7, 37–44.

Baxter, C., Poonia, K., Ward, L., and Nadirshaw, Z. (1990), *Double Discrimination: Issues and Services for People with Learning Disabilities from Black and Ethnic Minority Communities*, London: King's Fund.

Bayley, M. (1973), *Mental Handicap and Community Care: A Study of Mentally Handicapped People in Sheffield*, London: Routledge and Kegan Paul.

Bennett, A. (2005), *Untold Stories*, London: Faber and Faber/Profile Books.

Bersani, H. (1998), 'From Social Clubs to Social Movement: Landmarks in the Development of International Self-Advocacy Movement', in Ward (ed.) *Innovations in Advocacy and Empowerment*, pp. 59–76.

Berton, P. (1959), 'What's Wrong at Orillia: Out of Site Out of Mind', *Toronto Star*, 31 December.

Bigby, C. (2005), 'The Impact of Policy Tensions and Organizational Demands on the Process of Moving Out of an Institution', in Johnson and Traustadottir (eds), *Deinstitutionalisation and People with Intellectual Disabilities*, pp. 117–29.

Billis, D., and Glennerster, H. (1998), 'Human Services and the Voluntary Sector: Towards a Theory of Comparative Advantage', *Journal of Social Policy*, vol. 27, no. 1, 79–98.

Black Friendly Group (2004), *Telling It Ourselves: 'An Oral History'*, York: Joseph Rowntree Foundation.

Blatt, B., and Mangel, C. (1967), 'Tragedy and Hope of Retarded Children', *Look* 31, 31 October, 96–9.

Blunden, R. (1980), *Individual Plans for Mentally Handicapped People: A Draft Procedural Guide*, Cardiff: Mental Handicap in Wales Applied Research Unit, University of Wales College of Medicine.

Board of Education (1947), *Health of the School Child, 1939–45*, London: HMSO.

Board of Education and Board of Control (1929), *Report of the Mental Deficiency Committee*, Parts 1–IV, London: HMSO.

Booth, T., Simons, K., and Booth, W. (1990), *Outward Bound: Relocation and Community Care for People with Learning Difficulties*, Buckingham: Open University Press.

Bornat, J. (1992), 'The Communities of Community Publishing', *Oral History*, vol. 20, no. 2, 23–31.

Bornat, J. (2005), 'Buying Care and Assistance', Workbook 4, *K202 Care Welfare and Community* (2nd edn), Milton Keynes: Open University, pp. 105–52.

Borsay, A. (2005), *Disability and Social Policy in Britain Since 1750: A History of Exclusion*, Basingstoke: Palgrave Macmillan.

Boston, S. (1981), *Will, My Son*, London: Pluto Press.

Bourdieu, P. (1977), *Outline of a Theory of Practice*, Cambridge: Cambridge University Press.

Braddock, D. (1987), *Federal Policy Toward Mental Retardation and Developmental Disabilities*, Baltimore: Brookes.

Braddock, D., Hemp, R., Fujiura, G., Bachelder, L., and Mitchell, D. (1990), *The State of the States in Developmental Disabilities*, Baltimore: Brookes.

Brandon, D., and Ridley, J. (1985), *Beginning to Listen*, London: Campaign for People with Mental Handicaps.

Brandon, M. W. G. (1960), 'A Survey of 200 Women Discharged from a Mental Deficiency Hospital', *Journal of Mental Science*, vol. 106, 355–70.

Brechin, A., and Walmsley, J. (eds) (1989), *Making Connections: Reflecting on the Lives and Experiences of People with Learning Difficulties: A Reader*, London: Hodder and Stoughton.

Brenton, M. (1985), *The Voluntary Sector in British Social Service*, Harlow: Longman Group.

Bridgen, P., and Lowe, R. (1998), *Welfare Policy Under the Conservatives 1951–1964: A Guide to the Documents in the Public Record Office*, London: Public Record Office.

Brigham, L., Atkinson, D., Jackson, M., Rolph, S., and Walmsley, J. (eds) (2000), *Crossing Boundaries: Change and Continuity in the History of Learning Disability*, Kidderminster: BILD Publications.

British Psychological Society (2001), *Learning Disability: Definition and Contexts*, Leicester: British Psychological Society.

Brown, A., and Barrett, D. (2002), *Knowledge of Evil: Child Prostitution and Child Sexual Abuse in Twentieth Century England*, London: Wilan Publishing.

Brown, H., and Smith, H. (eds) (1992), *Normalisation: A Reader for the Nineties*, London: Routledge.

Brown, H., and Walmsley, J. (1997), 'When "Ordinary" isn't Enough: A Review of the Concept of Normalization', in J. Bornat *et al.* (eds), *Community Care: A Reader* (2nd edn), London: Macmillan, pp. 227–36.

Buck, P. S. (1950), *The Child that Never Grew*, New York: John Day.

Buchanan, I., and Walmsley, J. (2006), 'Self-Advocacy in Historical Perspective', *British Journal of Learning Disabilities*, vol. 34, no. 3, 133–8.

Bulmer, M. (1987), *The Social Basis of Community Care*, London: Unwin Hyman.

Burke, P., and Signo, C. (1996), *Support for Families*, Aldershot: Ashgate.

Burnside, M. (1991), *My Life Story*, Halifax: Pecket Well College.

Burt, C. (1952), *Mental and Scholastic Tests*, London: PS King.

Burton, M., and Kagan, C. (2006), 'Decoding *Valuing People*', *Disability and Society*, vol. 21, no. 4, 299–314.

Busfield, J. (1986), *Managing Madness: Changing Ideas and Practice*, London: Hutchinson.

Bylov, F. (2006), 'Patterns of Culture and Power After "The Great Release": The History of Movements of Subculture and Empowerment Among Danish People with Learning Difficulties', *British Journal of Learning Disabilities*, vol. 34, no. 3, pp. 139–45.

Bytheway, B., and Johnson, J. (1998), 'The Social Construction of "Carers" ', in A. Symonds and A. Kelly (eds), *The Social Construction of Community Care*, Basingstoke: Macmillan, pp. 241–53.

Bytheway, B., Bacigalupo, V., Bornat, J., Johnson, J., and Spurr, S. (eds) (2002), *Understanding Care, Welfare and Community: A Reader*, London: Routledge.

Cambridge, P., Hayes, L., and Knapp, M. (1993), *Care in the Community: Five Years On*, Aldershot: Ashgate.

Campbell, J., and McColgan, M. (2002), 'Social Work in Northern Ireland', in Payne and Shardlow (eds), *Social Work in the British Isles*, pp. 105–30.

Campbell, J., and Oliver, M. (1996), *Disability Politics: Understanding Our Past, Changing our Future*, Leeds: Disability Press, London: Routledge.

Caplan, G. (1961), *An Approach to Community Mental Health*, New York: Grune and Stratton.

Carter, J. (1981), *Day Services for Adults: Somewhere to Go*, London: George, Allen and Unwin.

Castell, J. H. F., and Mittler, P. J. (1965), 'Intelligence of Patients in Subnormality Hospitals: A Survey of Admissions in 1961', *British Journal of Psychiatry*, vol. 111, 219–25.

Cavalier, A. R., and McCarver, R. B. (1981), '*Wyatt v. Stickney* and Mentally Retarded Individuals', *Mental Retardation*, vol. XIX, 209–14.

Chapman, R. (2005), 'The Role of the Self-Advocacy Support-Worker in UK People First Groups: Developing Inclusive Research' (Open University Unpublished PhD thesis).

Chappell, A. L. (1992), 'Towards a Sociological Critique of the Normalisation Principle', *Disability, Handicap and Society*, vol. 7, no. 1, 35–51.

Chappell, A. L. (1997), 'From Normalization to Where?', in L. Barton and M. Oliver (eds), *Disability Studies: Past, Present and Future*, Leeds: Disability Press, pp. 45–61.

Charlton, J. (1998), *Nothing About Us Without Us: Disability, Oppression and Empowerment*, Berkeley, CA: University of California Press.

Christie, N., and Gauvreau, M. (eds) (2004), *Mapping the Margins: The Family and Social Discipline in Canada, 1700–1945*, Montreal: McGill-Queens University Press.

Chupik, J., and Wright, D. (2006), 'Treating the "Idiot" Child in early 20th-Century Ontario', *Disability and Society*, vol. 21, no. 1, 77–90.

Circular I-19/2000, *Status for Tilbudet til Mennesker Med Psykisk Utviklinghemming [State of the Services for People with Learning Disabilities]*, Oslo: Department of Social Affairs.

Clarke, A., and Clarke, A. D. B. (1972), 'Problems of Employment and Occupation of the Mentally Subnormal', in Adams and Lovejoy (eds), *The Mentally Subnormal: Social Work Approaches*, pp. 233–68.

Clarke, A. D. B., and Clarke, A. (1973), *Mental Retardation and Behavioural Research*, Edinburgh and London: Churchill Livingstone.

Clarke, A. D. B., and Clarke, A. M. (1953), 'How Constant is the IQ?', *Lancet*, vol. ii, 877–80.

Clarke, A. D. B., and Hermelin, B. F. (1955), 'Adult Imbeciles, Their Abilities and Trainability', *Lancet*, vol. ii, 337–9.

Clarke, A. M., and Clarke, A. D. B. (1958), *Mental Deficiency: The Changing Outlook* (1st edn), London: Methuen & Co.

Clarke, A. M., and Clarke, A. D. B. (1974), *Mental Deficiency: The Changing Outlook* (3rd edn), London: Methuen & Co.

Clement, T. (2004), 'An Anthropology of People First, Anytown' (Open University Unpublished PhD thesis).

Coalition Against Institutions as Community Resource Centres (1986), *Institutions: New Forms New Fears*.

Collins, J. (1992), *When the Eagles Fly*, London: Values into Action.

Collins, J. (1993), *The Resettlement Game*, London: Values into Action.

Collins, J. (1994), *Still to be Settled*, London: Values into Action.

Community Services Victoria (1989), *State Plan for Intellectual Disability Services*, Melbourne: Community Services Victoria.

Community Visitors (1990), *Annual Report of the Community Visitors 1990*, Melbourne: Office of the Public Advocate.

Concannon, L. (2004), *Planning for Life: Involving Adults with Learning Disabilities in Service Planning*, London: Routledge.

Cooper, M. (1997), 'Mabel Cooper's Life Story', in Atkinson, Jackson and Walmsley (eds), *Forgotten Lives*, pp. 21–34.

Cooper, M. (2000), 'My Quest to Find Out', in Atkinson *et al.* (eds), *Good Times, Bad Times*, pp. 184–8.

Coventry, M. (2000), 'Then and Now', in Atkinson *et al.* (eds), *Good Times, Bad Times*, pp. 193–6.

Cox, C., and Pearson, M. (1995), *Made to Care: The Case for Residential and Village Communities for People with a Mental Handicap*, London: Rannock Trust.

Cox, P. (1996), 'Girls, Deficiency and Delinquency', in Digby and Wright (eds), *From Idiocy to Mental Deficiency*, pp.184–206.

Craft, M. (1962), 'The Rehabilitation of the Imbecile: A Follow-Up Report', *British Journal of Mental Subnormality*, vol. 8, 26–7.

Craft, A. (ed.) (1987), *Mental Handicap and Sexuality: Issues and Perspectives*, Tunbridge Wells: Costello.

Crawley, B. (1989), *The Growing Voice*.

Crossley, N. (1998), 'Transforming the Mental Health Field: The Early History of the National Association for Mental Health', *Sociology of Health & Illness*, vol. 20, no. 4, 458–88.

Crossman, R. H. S. (1977), *The Diaries of a Cabinet Minister*, vol. 3, London: Hamish Hamilton and Jonathan Cape.

Crow, L. (1996), 'Including All of Our Lives: Reviewing the Social Model of Disability', in J. Morris (ed.), *Encounters with Strangers: Feminism and Disability*, London: Women's Press, pp. 206–26.

Dale, P. M. and Melling, J. (eds) (2006), *Mental Illness and Learning Disability Since 1850: Finding a Place for Mental Disorder in the United Kingdom*, London: Routledge.

Dalley, G. (1988), *Ideologies of Caring: Rethinking Community and Collectivism*, London: MacMillan.

Dalley, G. (1989), 'Community Care: The Ideal and the Reality', in Brechin and Walmsley (eds), *Making Connections*, pp. 199–208.

Davies, C., Hudson, B., and Hardy, B. (2005), 'Working Towards Partnership', Workbook 4, *K202 Care Welfare and Community* (2nd edn), Milton Keynes: Open University, pp. 59–104.

Davies, C. A., and Jenkins, R. (1997), 'She has Different Fits to Me: How People with Learning Difficulties See Themselves', *Disability and Society*, vol. 12, no. 1, 95–109.

Davis, K. (1999), 'The Disabled People's Movement: Putting the Power in Empowerment' in M. Barnes and L. Warren (eds), *Paths to Empowerment*, Bristol: Policy Press, pp. 15–24.

Deacon, J. J. (1974), *Tongue Tied: Fifty Years of Friendship in a Subnormality Hospital*, London: National Society for Mentally Handicapped Children.

Deal, M. (2003), 'Disabled People's Attitudes Toward Other Impairment Groups: A Hierarchy of Impairments', *Disability and Society*, vol. 18, no. 7, 897–910.

Dearden-Phillips, C., and Fountain, R. (2005), 'Real Power? An Examination of the Involvement of People with Learning Difficulties in Strategic Service Development in Cambridgeshire', *British Journal of Learning Disability*, vol. 33, no. 4, 200–4.

Dendy, M. (1903), 'The Feeble Minded', *Economic Review*, vol. 13, no. 3, 257–79.

Department of Human Services (2002), *State Disability Plan 2002–2012*, Melbourne: Department of Human Services.

Department of Human Services (2005a), *Strengthening and Building Participatory Practice*, Melbourne: Department of Human Services.

Department of Human Services (2005b), *Disability Action Planning: A Policy Framework for Victorian Government Departments*, Melbourne: Department of Human Services.

Department of Human Services (2005c), *MetroAccess: Building Inclusive Communities*, Melbourne: Department of Human Services.

Department of Human Services (2006), *Disability Bill: Exposure Draft*, Melbourne: Department of Human Services.

DES (1978), Committee of Enquiry into the Education of Handicapped Children and Young People, *Special Educational Needs: A Report* (Cmnd. 7212), London: HMSO.

DETR (1999), *DETR Circular 10/99: Local Government Act 1999: Part 1, Best Value*, London: DETR.

Deutsch, A. (1948), *The Shame of the States*, New York: Harcourt, Brace.

DfEE (1997), *Excellence for All Children*, London: HMSO.

DHSS (1968), *Report of the Committee on Local Authority and Allied Personal Social Services*, London: HMSO.

DHSS, Welsh Office (1971), *Better Services for the Mentally Handicapped* (Cmnd. 4683), London: HMSO.

DHSS (1975), *Better Services for the Mentally Ill* (Cmnd. 6233), London: HMSO.

DHSS (1980), *Mental Handicap: Progress, Problems and Priorities: A Review of Mental Handicap Services in England and Wales Since the 1971 White Paper 'Better Services for the Mentally Handicapped'*, London: HMSO.

DHSS (NI) (1991), *People First*, Belfast: HMSO.

Digby, A. (1989), *British Welfare Policy: Workhouse to Workfare*, London: Faber.

Digby, A., and Wright, D. (eds) (1996), *From Idiocy to Mental Deficiency: Historical Perspectives on People with Learning Difficulties*, London: Routledge.

Di Terlizzi, M. (1994), 'Life History: The Impact of a Changing Service Provision on an Individual with Learning Disabilities', *Disability and Society*, vol. 9, no. 4, 501–17.

DOH (1981a), *Care in the Community: A Consultative Document on Moving Resources for Care in England*, London: HMSO.

DOH (1981b), *Growing Older* (Cmnd. 8173), London: HMSO.

DOH (1989), *Caring for People – Community Care in the Next Decade and Beyond* (Cm. 849), London: HMSO.

DOH (2001a), *Valuing People: A New Strategy for Learning Disability for the 21st Century* (Cm. 5086), Norwich: The Stationery Office.

DOH (2001b), *Valuing People: Accessible Version*, Norwich: The Stationery Office.

DOH (2002), *Review of Mental Health and Learning Disabilities (Northern Ireland)*, available at http://www.rmhldni.gov.uk/

DOH (2005), *Independence, Well Being and Choice: Our Vision for the Future of Social Care Services for Adults in England* (Green Paper), London: Department of Health.

DOH (nd), *Valuing People: Towards Person Centred Approaches*, London: Department of Health.

Donges, G. (1982), *Policy Making for the Mentally Handicapped*, Aldershot: Gower.

Downer, J., and Ferns, P. (1998), 'Self-Advocacy by Black People with Learning Difficulties', in Ward (ed.), *Innovations in Advocacy and Empowerment for People with Intellectual Disabilities*, pp. 141–50.

Dumbleton (2005), 'On Being a Parent in the Twenty First Century', paper given at the Social History of Learning Disability Conference, Open University, Milton Keynes, 2005.

Edge, J. (2001), *Who's in Control? Decision-Making by People with Learning Difficulties who have high Support Needs*, London: Values Into Action.

Edwards, K. (1992), *Contracts in Practice: A Practical Guide for Voluntary Organisations*, London: NCVO/Directory of Social Change.

Emerson, E. (1992), 'What is Normalisation?', in Brown and Smith (eds), *Normalisation: A Reader for the Nineties*, pp. 1–18.

Emerson, E., Malam, S., Davies, I., and Spencer, K. (2005), *Adults with Learning Difficulties in England 2003/4*, London: Office of National Statistics.

Ericsson, K. (2002), *From Institutional Life to Community Participation*, Uppsala: University of Uppsala.

Ericsson, K., and Mansell, J. (1996), 'Introduction', in J. Mansell and K. Ericsson (eds), *Deinstitutionalisation and Community Living: Intellectual Disability Services in Britain, Scandinavia and the USA*, London: Chapman & Hall, pp. 1–16.

Esher, F. J. S. (1965), 'Subnormality Hostels: Two Different Functions', *Mental Health*, vol. 24, no. 3, 124–5.

Evans, G., Todd, S., Beyer, S., Felce, D., and Perry, J. (1994), 'Assessing the Impact of the All Wales Mental Handicap Strategy', *Journal of Intellectual Disability Research*, vol. 38, 109–33.

'Everybody's Business' (1961), *Spectator*, 17 March, pp. 351–2.

Fagan, N., and Plant, T. (2003), 'Joint Practitioners in Health and Social Care', in M. Jukes and M. Bollard (eds), *Contemporary Learning Disability Practice*, Wiltshire: Quay Books.

Faulkner, R. E. (1969), 'The Opportunity Class: A Pre-School Approach to the Handicapped Child', *Forward Trends*, November.

Fay, M., Morrisey, M., and Smyth, M. (1999), *The Cost of the Troubles*, London: Zed.

Felce, D., Grant, G., Todd, S., Ramcharan, P., McGrath, M., Perry, J., and Kilsby, M. (1998), *Towards a Full Life: Researching Policy Innovation for People With Learning Disabilities*, London: Butterworth-Heinemann.

Ferris, G. (1998), *My Life with Family and Friends*, Milton Keynes: Private Publication.

Finkelstein, V. (1980), *Attitudes and Disabled People: Issues for Discussion*, New York: World Rehabilitation Fund.

Finlay, W. M. L., and Lyons, E. (2000), 'Social Categorisations, Social Comparisons and Stigma: Presentations of Self in People with Learning Difficulties', *British Journal of Social Psychology*, vol. 39, 129–46.

Finlayson, G. (1990), 'A Moving Frontier: Voluntarism and the State in British Social Welfare 1941–1949', *Twentieth Century British History*, vol. 1, no. 2, 183–206.

Fisher, L. (2005), 'Why Us?' in Rolph *et al.* (eds), *Witnesses to Change*, pp. 87–94.

Flynn, M., and Ward, L. (1991), ' "We can Change the Future": Self and Citizen Advocacy', in S. Segal and V. Varma (eds), *Prospects for People with Learning Difficulties*, London: David Fulton, pp. 129–48.

Fox, E. (1940), 'Emergency Hostels for Difficult Children', *Mental Health*, vol. 1, no. 4, 97–102.

Fox, J. W. (1929), 'After Careers of the Feebleminded', *Medical Officer*, vol. 41, 251–2.

Freeman, H., and Farndale, J. (eds), *Trends in the Mental Health Services: A Symposium of Original and Reprinted Papers*, Oxford: Pergamon.

French, C. (1972), *A History of the Development of the Mental Health Service in Bedfordshire 1948–1970*, Bedford: Bedfordshire County Council Health Committee.

Fryson, R., and Ward, L. (eds) (2004), *Making Valuing People Work: Strategies for Change in Services for People with Learning Disabilities*, Bristol: Policy Press.

Fyfe, N. R., and Milligan, C. (2003), 'Out of the Shadows: Exploring Contemporary Geographies of Voluntarism', *Progress in Human Geography*, vol. 27, no. 4, 397–413.

Fyffe, C., McCubbery, J., Frawley, P., Laurie, D., and Bigby, C. (2004a), *Disability Advocacy Unit Model Development Report*, Melbourne: Disability Services Division, Department of Human Services.

Fyffe, C., McCubbery, J., Frawley, P., Laurie, D., and Bigby, C. (2004b), *Self Advocacy Resource Unit Model Development Report*, Melbourne: Disability Services Division, Department of Human Services.

Gabbay, J., and Webster, C. (1983), 'General Introduction: Changing Educational Provision for the Mentally Handicapped: From the 1890s to the 1980s', *Oxford Review of Education*, vol. 9, no. 3, 169–75.

Gehlbach, N. L. (2001), 'Lincoln State School: A Little History of a Big Place', *Our Times*, vol. 5, Winter, 3–5.

Gelb, S. (2004), 'Mental Deficients Fighting Fascism: The Unplanned Normalisation of World War II', in Noll and Trent (eds), *Mental Retardation in America*, pp. 308–21.

Gibson, F. (1998), *Reminiscence and Recall*, London: UK Age Concern Books.

Gibson, W. (1930), 'The Hostel Method for Feeble-Minded Young Men and Women', *Mental Welfare*, vol. 2, 75–7.

Gillman, M., Swain, J., and Heyman, B. (1997), 'Life History or Case History: The Objectification of People with Learning Difficulties Through the Tyranny of Professional Discourses', *Disability and Society*, vol. 12, no. 5, 675–93.

Glendinning, C. (1983), *Unshared Care: Parents and their Disabled Children*, London: Routledge and Kegan Paul.

Goffman, E. (1961), *Asylums: Essays on the Social Situation of Mental Patients and Other Inmates*, Harmondsworth: Penguin.

Goffman, E. (1963), *Stigma: Notes on the Management of Spoiled Identity*, Harmondsworth: Penguin.

Goodley, D. (1996), 'Tales of Hidden Lives: A Critical Examination of Life History Research with People who have Learning Difficulties', *Disability and Society*, vol. 11, no. 3, 333–48.

Goodley, D. (2000), *Self-Advocacy in the Lives of People with Learning Difficulties: The Politics of Resilience*, Buckingham: Open University Press.

Goodley, D. (2002), 'What's in a Label?', *Community Living*, vol. 15, no. 3, 2.

Graham, H. (1983), 'Caring: A Labour of Love', in J. Finch and D. Groves (eds), *A Labour of Love: Women, Work and Caring*, London: Routledge and Kegan Paul, pp. 13–30.

Grant, G., and Ramcharan, P. (eds) (2003), 'Valuing People – The Interface with Research', *British Journal of Learning Disabilities*, Special Issue, vol. 31, no. 4, 143–203.

Green, A. (2004), 'Individual Remembering and "Collective Memory": Theoretical Presuppositions and Contemporary Debates', *Oral History*, vol. 32, no. 2, 35–44.

Griffiths Report (1988), *Community Care, An Agenda for Action*, London: HMSO.

Grover, C., and Stewart, J. (1999), ' "Market Workfare": Social Security, Social Regulation and Competitiveness in the 1990s', *Journal of Social Policy*, vol. 28, no. 1, 73–96.

Grunewald, K. (2004), 'Sweden: Closing Down of Institutions for Intellectually Disabled People is Completed', *Scandinavian Journal of Disability Research*, vol. 6, 265–73.

Hadley, R., and Hatch, S. (1981), *Social Welfare and the Failure of the State: Centralised Social Services and Participatory Alternatives*, London: Allen and Unwin.

Hall Carpenter Archives (1989), *Walking after Midnight: Gay Men's Life Stories*, London: Routledge.

Hall, V., and Rolph, S. (2005), ' "I've Got my Freedom Now": Memories of Transitions Into and Out of Institutions, 1932 to the Present Day' in Johnson and Traustadottir (eds), *Deinstitutionalisation and People with Intellectual Disabilities*, pp. 163–70.

Ham, C. (1981), *Policy-Making in the National Health Service: A Case Study of the Leeds Regional Hospital Board*, London: Macmillan.

Hannam, C. (1975), *Parents and Mentally Handicapped Children*, Harmondsworth: Penguin.

Hardy, D. (2005), 'Our Life with Margaret', in Rolph, *et al.* (eds), *Witnesses to Change*, pp. 41–5.

Hearn, J. (2000), *Claiming Scotland: National Identity and Liberal Culture*, Edinburgh: Polygan.

Hebden, J. (1985), *'She'll Never Do Anything, Dear'*, London: Souvenir Press.

Hechter, M. (1975), *Internal Colonialism: The Celtic Fringe in British National Development 1536–1966*, London: Routledge and Kegan Paul.

Hellan, B. (1992), *Hallsetheimen Personalforening. Historisk Tilbakeblikk 1935–1991* [*Hallsetheimen Union 1935–1991*], Klæbu: Hallsetheimen Personalforening.

Henderson, R., and Pochin, M. (2001), *A Right Result? Advocacy, Justice and Empowerment*, Bristol: Policy Press.

Herd, H. (1930), *The Diagnosis of Mental Deficiency*, London: Hodder and Stoughton.

Hersov, J. (1996), 'The Rise of Self-Advocacy in Great Britain' in G. Dybwad and H. Bersani (eds), *New Voices: Self-advocacy by People with Learning Disabilities*, pp. 130–9.

HMT (2002), *The Role of the Voluntary and Community Sector in Service Delivery: A Cross Cutting Review*, London: HMT.

House of Commons (1985), *Second Report from the Social Services Committee, Session 1984–1985. Community Care with Special Reference to Adults Mentally Ill and Mentally Handicapped People*, vol. 1, London: HMSO.

Howard, A. (1991), *Crossman: The Pursuit of Power* (Pimlico edn), London: Jonathan Cape.

Hubert, J. (1991), *Homebound: Crisis in the Care of Young People with Severe Learning Difficulties: A Story of 20 Families*, London: King's Fund Centre.

Humphries, S., and Gordon, P. (1992), *Out of Sight: The Experience of Disability 1900–1950*, Plymouth: Northcote House.

Hunt, N. (1967), *The World of Nigel Hunt*, Beaconsfield: Darwen Finlayson.

Hunter, D., and Wistow, G. (1987), *Community Care in Britain: Variations on a Theme*, London: King Edward's Hospital Fund.

Hutchinson, C. X. Jr (1946), 'It's Different in Connecticut', *Christian Century*, vol. LXIII, 241–2.

Intellectual Disability Services Task Force (1995), *Report to the Hon. Michael John, MP Minister for Community Services*, Melbourne: Health and Community Services.

Jackson, M. (2001), *The Borderland of Imbecility: Medicine, Society, and the Fabrication of the Feeble Mind in Late Victorian and Edwardian England*, Manchester: Manchester University Press.

'Jean' (2002), 'Out in the World', in Bytheway *et al.* (eds), *Understanding Care, Welfare and Community*, pp. 205–8.

Jessop, B. (1994), 'The Transition to Post-Fordism and the Schumpeterian Workfare State', in R. Burrow and B. Loader (eds), *Towards a Post-Fordist Welfare State?*, London: Routledge, pp. 13–37.

Jewish Women in London Group (1989), *Generations of Memories: Voices of Jewish Women*, London: Women's Press.

Johnson, J. (2005), 'Funding Matters', Workbook 4, *K202 Care Welfare and Community* (2nd edn), Milton Keynes: Open University, pp. 7–57.

Johnson, K. (1998), *Deinstitutionalising Women: An Ethnographic Study of Institutional Closure*, Melbourne: Cambridge University Press.

Johnson, K., and Traustadottir, R. (eds) (2005), *Deinstitutionalisation and People with Intellectual Disabilities: In and Out of Institutions*, London: Jessica Kingsley.

Jones, G. (1986), *Social Hygiene in Twentieth Century Britain*, London: Croom Helm.

Jones, K. (1954), 'Problems of Mental After-Care in Lancashire', *Sociological Review*, vol. 2, 34–56.

Jones, K. (1960), *Mental Health and Social Policy, 1845–1959*, London: Routledge and Kegan Paul.

Jones, K. (1975), *Opening the Door: A Study of New Policies for the Mentally Handicapped*, London: Routledge and Kegan Paul.

Jones, K. W. (2004), 'Education for Children with Mental Retardation: Parent Activism, Public Policy and Family Ideology in the 1950s', in Noll and Trent (eds), *Mental Retardation in America*, pp. 322–50.

JRF (2002), *Fulfilling the Promises: A Response from the Joseph Rowntree Foundation to the Proposed Framework for Services for People with Learning Disabilities in Wales*, York: JRF. Available at www.jrf.org.uk/knowledge/responses/docs/learningdisabilitesinwales.asp

JRF (2005), *Monitoring Poverty and Social Exclusion in Scotland 2005*, York: JRF. Available at www.jrf.org.uk/knowledge/findings/social policy/0585.asp

Judge, C., and van Brummelen, F. (2002), *Kew Cottages: The World of Dolly Stainer*, Melbourne: Spectrum Publications.

Kendal, J., and Knapp, M. (1996), *The Voluntary Sector in the UK*, Manchester: Manchester University Press.

Kerby, P. (1967), 'The Reagan Backlash: Revolt against the Poor,' *Nation*, vol. CCV, 25 November, 262–7.

Kesey, K. (1962), *One Flew Over the Cuckoo's Nest*, New York: Viking.

Kestenbaum, A. (1996), *Independent Living: A Review*, York: Joseph Rowntree Foundation.

Kevles, D. J. (1995), *In the Name of Eugenics: Genetics and the Uses of Human Heredity* (revised edn), New York: Alfred A. Knopf.

Kiely, R., Bechofer, F., and McCrone, D. (2005), 'Birth, Blood and Belonging: Identity Claims in Post Devolution Scotland', *Sociological Review*, vol. 53, no. 1, 150–71.

King, D. (1999), *In the Name of Liberalism: Illiberal Social Policy in the United States and Britain*, Oxford: Oxford University Press.

King's Fund (1980), *An Ordinary Life*, London: King's Fund.

King's Fund Centre (1988), *Ties and Connections: An Ordinary Community Life for People with Learning Difficulties*, London: King's Fund Centre.

Kollings, P. E. (1962), 'Story of a Father and Mother Who Have Solved the Most Perplexing Problem Parents Can Face', *Better Homes and Gardens*, vol. XL, 56–7.

Krause, A., and Stolzfus, G. M. (1948), *Forgotten Children: The Story of Mental Deficiency*, Philadelphia, PA: National Mental Health Foundation.

Kugel, R. B., and Shearer, A. (1976), *Changing Patterns in Residential Services for the Mentally Retarded* (revised edn), Washington: US Government Printing Office.

Kushlick, A. (1969), 'Care of the Mentally Subnormal', *Lancet*, vol. ii, 1196–7.

Kushlick, A. (1974), 'The Need for Residential Care', in D. M. Boswell and J. M. Wingrove (eds), *The Handicapped Person in the Community*, London: Tavistock Publications/Open University Press, pp. 307–17.

Laing and Buisson (1998, 1999), *Care of Elderly People: Market Survey* (10th and 11th edns), London: Laing and Buisson.

Langness, H. G., and Levine (1986), *Culture and Retardation: Life Histories of Mildly Mentally Retarded Persons in American Society*, Boston, MA: D. Reidel Publishing Company.

Lapage, C. P. (1911), *Feeblemindedness in Children of School Age*, Manchester: Manchester University Press.

Larsson, S., and Lakin, C. (1991), 'Parents' Attitudes about Residential Placement before and after Deinstitutionalisation', *Journal of the Association of People with Severe Handicaps*, vol. 14, 24–38.

Lasch, C. (1995), *The Revolt of the Elites and the Betrayal of Democracy*, New York: W.W. Norton and Co.

Lerman, P. (1982), *Deinstitutionalization and the Welfare State*, New Brunswick, NJ: Rutgers University Press.

Leslie, I. M. (1939–41), 'Some Problems of a Hostel in a Reception Area', *Social Work*, vol. 1, 307–12.

Lewis, J. (1995a), *The Voluntary Sector, the State and Social Work in Britain*, Aldershot: Edward Elgar.

Lewis, J. (1995b), 'Family Provision of Health and Welfare in the Mixed Economy of Care in the Late Nineteenth and Twentieth Centuries', *Social History of Medicine*, vol. 8, no. 1, 1–16.

Lord, J. (1985), *Creating Responsive Communities*, Toronto: OAMR.

Lovejoy, H. (1972), 'Community Hostels', in Adams and Lovejoy (eds), *The Mentally Subnormal: Social Work Approaches*, pp. 220–8.

Lowe, R. (2003), 'Education, 1900–1939', in C. Wrigby (ed.), *A Companion to Early Twentieth Century Britain*, Oxford: Blackwell, pp. 424–37.

Lowe, R. (2005), *The Welfare State in Britain since 1945* (3rd edn), London: Macmillan.

Lyons, J. F., and Heaton-Ward, W. A. (1955), *Notes on Mental Deficiency* (3rd edn), Bristol: John Wright and Sons.

Macnicol, J. (1987), 'In Pursuit of the Underclass', *Journal of Social Policy*, vol. 16, no. 3, 293–318.

Macnicol, J. (1989), 'Eugenics and the Campaign for Voluntary Sterilization in Britain Between the Wars', *Social History of Medicine*, vol. 2, no. 2, 147–70.

Mairs, N. (1986), 'On Being a Cripple', in *Plaintexts: Essays, 9–20*, Tucson: University of Arizona Press.

Malin, N., Race, D., and Jones, G. (1980), *Services for the Mentally Handicapped in Britain*, London: Croom Helm.

Malster, R. (1994), *St Lawrence's: The Story of a Hospital, 1870–1994*, Caterham: Lifecare NHS Trust.

Marcus, A. D. (2005), 'Eli's Choice', *The Wall Street Journal*, vol. CCXLVI, 31 December, A1, A6.

Marks, D. (1999), *Disability: Controversial Debates and Psychosocial Perspectives*, London: Routledge.

Marquand, D. (1988), *The Unprincipled Society: New Demands and Old Politics*, London: Fontana Press.

Martin, F. M. (1984), *Between the Acts: Community Mental Health Services 1959–1983*, London: Nuffield Provincial Hospitals Trust.

McAndrew, C., and Edgerton, R. (1964), 'The Everyday Life of the Institutionalised "Idiots",' *Human Organization*, vol. 23, 312–18.

McCarthy, M. (1998), 'Sexual Violence Against Women with Learning Disabilities', *Feminism and Psychology*, vol. 8, no. 4, 544–51.

McConkey, R. (2005), 'Multi-Agency Working', *Journal of Intellectual Disabilities*, vol. 9, no. 3, 193–207.

McCormack, M. (1978), *A Mentally Handicapped Child in the Family*, London: Constable.

McWhorter, A., and Kappel, B. (1984), *Mandate For Quality, Vol. II Missing the Mark: An Analysis of the Ontario Government's Five Year Plan*, Toronto: NIMR.

Means, R., and Smith, R. (1985), *The Development of Welfare Services for Elderly People*, London: Croom Helm.

Means, R., and Smith, R. (1994), *Community Care: Policy and Practice*, Basingstoke: Macmillan.

Means, R., Richards, S., and Smith, R. (2003), *Community Care: Policy and Practice* (3rd edn), London: Palgrave.

Melling, J., Adair and Forsythe, W. (1997), 'A Proper Lunatic for Two Years: Pauper Lunatic Children in Victorian and Edwardian England: Child Admissions to Devon County Asylum, 1845–1914', *Journal of Social History*, Winter, 370–405.

Mercer, J. R. (1972), 'IQ: The Lethal Label', *Psychology Today*, vol. VI, September, 44–7, 95–7.

Metzel, D. (2004), 'Historical Social Geography', in Noll and Trent (eds) *Mental Retardation in America*, pp. 420–44.

Ministry of Health (1951), *Report of the Committee on Social Workers in the Mental Health Services* (Cmd. 8260), London: HMSO.

Ministry of Health (1962), *A Hospital Plan for England and Wales* (Cmnd. 1604), London: HMSO.

Ministry of Health (1963), *Health and Welfare: The Development of Community Care: Plans for the Health and Welfare Services of the Local Authorities in England and Wales* (Cmnd. 1973), London: HMSO.

Ministry of Health, Department of Health for Scotland (1959), *Report of the Working Party on Social Workers in the Local Authority Health and Welfare Services*, London: HMSO.

Ministry of Labour and National Service (1956), *Report of the Committee of Inquiry on the Rehabilitation, Training, and Resettlement of Disabled Persons* (Cmd. 9883), London: HMSO.

Mir, G., Nocon, A., Ahmad, W., with Jones, L. (2001), *Learning Difficulties and Ethnicity: Report to the Department of Health*, London: DOH.

Mitchell, D. (2000), 'Ambiguous Boundaries: Retrieving the History of Learning Disability Nursing', in Brigham *et al.* (eds), *Crossing Boundaries*, pp. 123–34.

Mitchell, D, Traustadottir, R., Chapman, R., Townson, L., Ingham, N., and Ledger, S. (eds) (2006), *Exploring Experiences of Advocacy by People with Learning Difficulties: Testimonies of Resistance*, London: Jessica Kingsley.

Mitchell, P. (1999), 'Self-Advocacy and Families' (Unpublished PhD thesis, Open University).

Mittler, P. (1966), *The Mental Health Services*, London: Fabian Society.

Mittler, P. (1996), 'Advocates and Advocacy', in P. Mittler and V. Sinason (eds), *Changing Policy and Practice for People with Learning Disabilities*, London: Cassell.

Mittler, P., and Castell, J. H. F. (1964), 'Hospital and Community Care of the Subnormal', *Lancet*, vol. i, 873–5.

Mittler, P., and Woodward, M. (1966), 'The Education of Children in Hospitals for the Subnormal: A Survey of Admissions', *Developmental Medicine and Child Neurology*, vol. 8, 16–25.

Mohan, J. (2002), *Planning, Markets and Hospitals*, London: Routledge.

Moore, M. (2004), 'The Death Story of David Hope' in D. Goodley *et al.* (eds), *Researching Life Stories: Method, Theory and Analyses in a Biographical Age*, London: Routledge/Falmer, pp. 26–39.

Morley, K. (1973), 'Industrial Training – Problems and Implications', in Clarke and Clarke (eds), *Mental Retardation and Behavioural Research*, pp. 125–30.

Moroney, R. M. (1976), *The Family and the State: Considerations for Social Policy*, London: Longman.

Morris, J. (1993a), *Independent Lives? Community Care and Disabled People*, London: Macmillan.

Morris, J. (1993b), *Community Care or Independent Living*, York: Joseph Rowntree Foundation in association with *Community Care*.

Morris, J. (2004), 'Independent Living and Community Care: A Disempowering Framework', *Disability and Society*, vol. 19, no. 5, 427–42.

Morris, P. (1969), *Put Away: A Sociological Study of Institutions for the Mentally Retarded*, London: Routledge and Kegan Paul.

Moscovitch, A., and Drover, G. (1987), 'Social Expenditures and the Welfare State: The Canadian Experience in Historical Perspective', in A. Moscovitch and J. Albert (eds), *The Benevolent State: The Growth of Welfare in Canada*, Toronto: Garamond Press, pp. 13–43.

Naufal, R. (1989), 'The Ten Year Plan for the Redevelopment of Intellectual Disability Services', *Policy Issues Forum*, April, 21–7.

Neilson Associates (1987a), *Ten Year Plan for the Redevelopment of Intellectual Disability Services. Interim Report. Part 1. The Form of the Task*, Melbourne: Community Services Victoria.

Neilson Associates (1987b), *Ten Year Plan for the Redevelopment of Intellectual Disability Services. Interim Report. Part 2. Quantification of the Task*, Melbourne: Community Services Victoria.

Neilson Associates (1988), *Ten Year Plan for the Redevelopment of Intellectual Disability Services. Final Report*, Melbourne: Community Services Victoria.

Nickson, B. (2005), 'Never Take no for an Answer' in Rolph *et al.* (eds), *Witnesses to Change*, pp. 77–86.

Nirje, B. (1969), 'The Normalization Principle and its Human Management Implications', in R. B. Kugel and W. Wolfensburger (eds), *Changing Patterns in Residential Services for the Mentally Retarded*, Washington, DC: Presidential Committee on Mental Retardation, pp. 231–52.

Nirje, B. (1970), 'The Normalisation Principle – Implications and Comments', *Journal of Mental Subnormality*, vol. 16, 62–70.

Noll, S., and Trent, J. W. Jr (eds) (2004), *Mental Retardation in America: A Historical Reader*, New York: New York University Press.

NOU (Norway's Public Committee Reports) (1973), no. 25, *Omsorg for Psykisk Utviklingshemmede* [*Services for Learning Disabled*], Oslo.

NOU (Norway's Public Committee Reports) (1985), no. 34, *Levekår for Utviklingshemmede* [*Level of Living for Learning Disabled*], Oslo.

NSMHCA (nd), *The NSMHC National Hostel and Sheltered Workshop*, London: NSMHCA.

OACL (1987a), *Alternatives to Institutions*, Toronto: OACL.
OACL (1987b), *Homes for Special Care and Nursing Homes: Relocating People to Homes in the Community*, Toronto: OACL.
OACL (nd), *Critical Review of 'Challenges and Opportunities': Community Living For People With Developmental Handicaps*, Toronto: OACL.
O'Brien, J. (1982), *Building Creative Tension: The Development of a Citizen Advocacy Program for People with Mental Handicaps*, Georgia, GA: Georgia Advocacy Office.
O'Brien, J., and Lyle, C. (1987), *Frameworks for Accomplishments: A Workshop for People Developing Better Services*, Decatur, GA: Responsive Systems Associates.
O'Brien, J., and Towell, D. (2003), 'Person Centred Planning in its Strategic Context: Towards a Framework for Reflection in Action', *Retrieved*, 29 May 2005.
O'Connor, N., and Tizard , J. (1954), 'A Survey of Patients in Twelve Mental Deficiency Institutions', *British Medical Journal*, vol. i, 16–18.
O'Connor, N., and Tizard, J. (1956), *The Social Problem of Mental Deficiency*, London: Pergamon Press.
Oettinger, K. B. (1963), 'Opening Doors for the Retarded Child', *New York Times Magazine*, 12 May, 68–9.
Office of the Public Advocate (1990), *Annual Report*, Melbourne: Office of the Public Advocate.
Oldham, J. (2004), *Sic Evenit Ratio Ut Componitur: The Little Book About Large System Change*, London: Kingsham Press.
Oliver, M. (1983), *Social Work and Disabled People*, Basingstoke: Macmillan.
Oliver, M. (1990), *The Politics of Disability*, London: Macmillan.
Oliver, M. (2004), 'Introduction', in J. Swain, S. French, C. Barnes and C. Thomas (eds), *Disabling Barriers: Enabling Environments* (2nd edn), London: Sage, pp. 1–4.
Ontario, ComSoc (1987), *Challenges and Opportunities: Community Living For People With Developmental Disabilities*, Toronto: ComSoc.
Ontario ComSoc (1988), *Transitions: Report of the Social Assistance Review Committee*, Toronto: ComSoc.
Ontario Office of Disabled Persons (1988), *Guide to Ontario Government Program and Services for Disabled Persons*, Toronto: Ontario Office of Disabled Persons.
Ontario, Provincial Secretariat for Social Development (1973), *Community Living For the Mentally Retarded: A New Policy Focus*, Toronto: Provincial Secretariat for Social Development.
Oswin, M. (1971), *The Empty Hours*, Harmondsworth: Penguin.
Oswin, M. (2000), 'Revisiting "The Empty Hours" ', in Brigham *et al.* (eds) *Crossing Boundaries*, pp. 135–45.
Owen, K. (2004), *'Going Home?': A Study of Women with Severe Learning Disabilities Moving out of a Locked Ward*, London: The Judith Trust.
Parents Voice (1969–87), London: NSMHC.
Payne, M., and Shardlow, S. (eds) (2002), *Social Work in the British Isles*, London: Jessica Kingsley.
Payne, S. (1969), 'Where Handicapped Mix with the Rest', *Times Educational Supplement*, 23 May 1969, 1712.
People First (1993), *Oi, it's my Assessment*, London: People First London Boroughs.
Pilgrim, D., and Rogers, A. (1993), *A Sociology of Mental Health and Illness*, Buckingham: Open University Press.

Plummer, K. (1983), *Documents of Life: An Introduction to the Problems and Literature of a Humanistic Method*, London: George Allen and Unwin.

Plummer, K. (2001), *Documents of Life 2: An Invitation to a Critical Humanism*, London: Sage Publications.

Potts, M., and Fido, R. (1991), *A Fit Person to be Removed: Personal Accounts of Life in a Mental Deficiency Institution*, Plymouth: Northcote House.

Priestley, M. (1999), *Disabled Politics and Community Care*, London: Jessica Kingsley.

Prochaska, F. (1988), *The Voluntary Impulse: Philanthropy in Modern Britain*, London: Faber and Faber.

Putnam, R. D. (2000), *Bowling Alone: The Collapse and Revival of American Community*, New York: Simon and Schuster.

'Question of Priorities' (1967), *Nation*, vol. CCV, 20 November, 516.

Race, D. (1999), *Social Role Valorisation and the English Experience*, London: Whiting and Birch.

Race, D., Boxall, K., and Carson, I. (2005), 'Towards a Dialogue for Practice: Reconciling Social Role Valorization with the Social Model of Disability', *Disability and Society*, vol. 20, no. 3, 507–22.

Ramcharan, P., Roberts, G., Grant, G., and Borland, J. (eds) (1997), *Empowerment in Everyday Life: Learning Disability*, London: Jessica Kingsley.

Rasmussen, M. (1962), En Tiårs Periode Innen åndssvakeomsorgen [Ten Years in Services for Mentally Retarded], *Hjertebladet*, vol. 2, 5–9.

Raynes, N., and King, R. (1972), 'Residential Care for the Mentally Retarded', in M. Boswell and J. Wingrove (eds), *The Handicapped Person in the Community*, London: Tavistock Publications/Open University Press.

Report of the Committee of Enquiry into Mental Handicap Nursing and Care (Cmnd. 7468), London: HMSO.

Report of the Committee of Inquiry into Allegations of Ill-Treatment of Patients and other Irregularities at the Ely Hospital, Cardiff (Cmnd. 3975), London: HMSO.

Report of the Royal Commission on the Care and Control of the Feeble-Minded (1908) (Cd. 4202), London: HMSO.

Ringsby Jansson, B. (2002), *Vardagslivets Arenor* [*Arenas of Everyday Life*], Gothenborg: Gothenborgs University.

Rioux, M., Bach, M., and Crawford, C. (1997), 'Citizenship and People with Disabilities in Canada: Towards the Elusive Ideal', in P. Ramcharan, G. Roberts, G. Grant, and J. Borland (eds), *Empowerment in Everyday Life: Learning Disability*, London: Jessica Kingsley, pp. 204–21.

Rivera, G. (1972), *Willowbrook: A Report on How It Is and Why It Doesn't Have To Be That Way*, New York: Random House.

Robb, B. (1967), *Sans Everything: A Case to Answer*, London: Nelson.

Roberts, C. A. (1963), *A Report on Ontario's Mental Health Services*, Ontario: Department of Health, Report of the Inter-Departmental Committee on Mental Retardation.

Rodgers, B. N., and Dixon, J. (1960), *Portrait of Social Work: A Study of Social Services in a Northern Town*, London: Oxford University Press for the Nuffield Provincial Hospitals Trust.

Roeher, G. A. (1976), 'ComServ', in Kugel and Shearer (eds), *Changing Patterns in Residential Services*, pp. 313–23.

Rogers, D. E. (1953), *Angel Unaware*, Westwood, NJ: Revell.

Rolph, S. (1999), 'Enforced Migrations by People with Learning Difficulties: A Case Study', *Oral History*, vol. 27, no. 1, 47–56.

Rolph, S. (2000), 'The History of Community Care for People with Learning Difficulties in Norfolk 1930–1980: The Role of Two Hostels' (Open University Unpublished PhD thesis).

Rolph, S. (2002), *Reclaiming the Past: The Role of Local Mencap Societies in the Development of Community Care in East Anglia, 1946–1980*, Milton Keynes: Open University.

Rolph, S. (2005a), *Building Bridges into the Community: The History of Bedford and District Society for People with Learning Disabilities, 1955–1990*, Milton Keynes: Open University.

Rolph, S. (2005b), *A New Voice: The History of South Norfolk Mencap Society 1974–1990*, Milton Keynes: Open University.

Rolph, S. (2005c), *Captured on Film: The History of Norwich and District Mencap Society 1954–1990*, Milton Keynes: Open University.

Rolph, S. (2005d), *Taking to the Stage: The History of Great Yarmouth and District Mencap Society 1969–1990*, Milton Keynes: Open University.

Rolph, S. (2005e), *'A Little Glamour with a Strict Tempo': The History of Cambridge Mencap Volume 1, 1947–1990*, Milton Keynes: Open University.

Rolph, S. (2005f), *'A Place in the Sun': The History of Lowestoft and District Mencap Society, 1962–1990*, Milton Keynes: Open University.

Rolph, S., and Walmsley, J. (2006), 'Oral History and New Orthodoxies: Narrative Accounts in the History of Learning Disability', *Oral History*, vol. 34, no. 1, 81–91.

Rolph, S., Atkinson, D., Nind, M., and Welshman, J. (2005), *Witnesses to Change: Families, Learning Difficulties and History*, Kidderminster: BILD Publications.

Rolph, S., Atkinson, D., and Walmsley, J. (2003), ' "A Pair of Stout Shoes and an Umbrella": The Role of the Mental Welfare Officer in Delivering Community Care in East Anglia: 1946–1970', *British Journal of Social Work*, vol. 33, no. 3, 339–59.

Rolph, S., Walmsley, J., and Atkinson, D. (2002), ' "A Man's Job"?: Gender Issues and the Role of Mental Welfare Officers, 1948–1970', *Oral History*, vol. 30, no. 1, 28–41.

Rooff, M. (1957), *Voluntary Societies and Social Policy*, London: Routledge and Kegan Paul.

Rose, J. (1995), 'Stress and Residential Staff: Towards an Integration of Existing Research', *Mental Handicap Research*, vol. 8, no. 4, 220–36.

Royal Commission on the Law Relating to Mental Illness and Mental Deficiency 1954–1957 (1957) (Cmnd. 169), London: HMSO.

Ryan, J., with Thomas, F. (1987), *The Politics of Mental Handicap* (revised edn), London: Free Association Books.

Sainsbury Centre for Mental Health (2005), *Beyond the Water Towers: The Unfinished Revolution in Mental Health Services 1985–2005*, London: Sainsbury Centre.

Sanctuary, G. (1981), *After I'm Gone: What will Happen to my Handicapped Child?* London: Souvenir Press.

Sanderson, H. (1998), 'A Say in My Future – Involving People with Profound and Multiple Disabilities in Person Centred Planning', in Ward (ed.), *Innovations in Advocacy and Empowerment*, pp. 161–81.

Sanderson, H. (2000), *Person Centred Planning: Key Features and Approaches*. Available at http://www.valuingpeople.gov.uk

Sanderson, H., Kennedy, J., Ritchie P., and Goodwin, G. (2002), *People, Plans and Possibilities*, Edinburgh: SHS.

Saxon-Harrold, S., and Kendall, J. (eds) (1993), *Researching the Voluntary Sector*, Tonbridge: Charities Aid Foundation.

Schwartzenberg, S. (2005), *Becoming Citizens: Family Life and the Politics of Disability*, Seattle and London: University of Washington Press.

Schweitzer, P. (1993), *Age Exchanges: Reminiscence Projects for Children and Older People*, London: Age Exchange.

Scottish Executive (2000), *The Same As You: A Review of Services for People with Learning Disabilities*, Edinburgh: The Stationery Office.

Scottish Executive (2004), *National Implementation Group: Report of the Short Life Working Group on Hospital Closure and Service Reprovision*, Edinburgh: The Stationery Office.

Scull, A. (1984), *Decarceration: Community Treatment and the Deviant – A Radical View* (second edn), Cambridge: Polity Press.

Searle, G. R. (1981), 'Eugenics and Class', in C. Webster (ed.), *Biology, Medicine and Society, 1840–1940*, Cambridge: Cambridge University Press, pp. 217–42.

Sedgwick, P. (1982), *Psycho Politics*, London: Pluto Press.

Shah, R. (1992), *The Silent Minority: Children with Disabilities in Asian Families*, London: National Children's Bureau.

Shakespeare, T. (2003), 'Having Come so Far, Where to Now?', *Times Higher Education Supplement*, 7 November, 28.

Shakespeare, T., Gillespie-Sells, K., and Davies, D. (1996), *The Sexual Politics of Disability: Untold Desires*, London: Cassell.

Shearer, A. (1986), *Building Community with People with Mental Handicaps, their Families and Friends*, London: King's Fund and CMH.

Shennan, V. (1980), *Our Concern: The Story of the National Association for Mentally Handicapped Children and Adults 1946–1980*, London: The National Association for Mentally Handicapped Adults and Children.

Shriver, E. K. (1962), 'Hope for Retarded Children', *Saturday Evening Post*, vol. CCXXXV, 71–5.

Shuttleworth, G. E., and Potts, W. A. (1910), *Mentally Deficient Children: Their Treatment and Training*, London: H. K. Lewis.

Simmons, H. (1982), *From Asylum To Welfare*, Toronto: National Institute on Mental Retardation.

Simons, K. (1992), *Sticking up for Yourself: Self Advocacy and People with Learning Difficulties*, York: Joseph Rowntree Foundation.

Simons, K. (1999), *A Place at the Table?*, Kidderminster: BILD Publications.

Sinason, V. (1992), *Mental Handicap and the Human Condition*, London: Free Association Books.

Sinclair, I. (1975), 'The Influence of Wardens and Matrons on Probation Hostels: A Study of a Quasi-Family Institution', in Tizard, Sinclair and Clarke (eds), *Varieties of Residential Experience*, pp. 122–40.

Sinclair, I. (ed.) (1988), *Residential Care: The Research Reviewed (Literature Surveys Commissioned by the Independent Review of Residential Care Chaired by Gillian Wagner)*, London: HMSO.

Sinson, J. (1993), *Group Homes and Integration of Developmentally Disabled People*, London: Jessica Kingsley.

Skouen, A. (1969), *De Veldedige Politikerne [Politics and Charity]*, Oslo: Aschehoug.

SOU (1981), no. 26, *Omsorger om Vissa Handikappade* [Services for Certain Disabled Groups], Stockholm.

Stainton, T. (1992), 'The Seeds of Change', *Community Living*, April, 20–2.

Stainton, T. (2000), 'Equal Citizens: The Discourse of Liberty and Rights in the History of Learning Disabilities', in Brigham *et al.* (eds) *Crossing Boundaries*, pp. 87–101.

Stewart, J. (2003), *Taking Stock: Scottish Social Welfare Since Devolution*, Bristol: Policy Press.

Stirling, N. (1983), *Pearl Buck: A Woman in Conflict*, Piscataway, NJ: New Century Publishers.

Strait, S. H. (1962), 'Bringing Up a Retarded Child', *Parents' Magazine*, vol. XXXVII, 51–3.

Strong, M. Kirkpatrick (1930), *Public Welfare Administration in Canada*, Chicago, IL: University of Chicago Press.

Swindon People First Research Team (2002), *Journey to Independence: Direct Payments for People with Learning Difficulties: Report to BILD*, Swindon: Swindon People First.

Szasz, T. (1961), *The Myth of Mental Illness*, New York: Harper and Row.

Taylor, F. (2006), 'Terms and Conditions', *Community Care*, 12–18 January, 38–9.

Taylor, M., and Lansley, J. (1992), 'Ideology and Welfare in the UK: The Implications for the Voluntary Sector', *Voluntas*, vol. 3, no. 2, 153–74.

Temby, E. (2005), 'Rowan's Choices', in Johnson and Traustadottir (eds), *Deinstitutionalization and People with Intellectual Disabilities*, pp. 117–44.

Tennyson, A. (1986), 'The Lady of Shalott', in J. Wain (ed.), *The Oxford Library of English Poetry*, Oxford: Oxford University Press, pp. 79–83.

Thomson, M. (1996), 'Family, Community, and State: The Micro-Politics of Mental Deficiency', in Digby and Wright (eds), *From Idiocy to Mental Deficiency*, pp. 207–30.

Thomson, M. (1998a), *The Problem of Mental Deficiency: Eugenics, Democracy, and Social Policy in Britain c.1870–1959*, Oxford: Clarendon Press.

Thomson, M. (1998b), 'Community Care and the Control of Mental Defectives in Inter-War Britain', in P. Horden and R. Smith (eds), *The Locus of Care: Families, Communities, Institutions and the Provision of Welfare Since Antiquity*, London: Routledge, pp. 176–97.

Thorne, D. (2005), *Goodbye all the Nurses*, Milton Keynes: Private Publication.

Tideman, M. (2000), *Normalisering och Kategorisering* [*Normalisation and Categorisation*], Stockholm: Johansson & Skyttmo Förlag.

Tideman, M. (2004). 'Socialt eller isolerad Integrerad? Om Institutionsavveckling och Integrering' ['Social Integration or Isolation? On Deinstitutionalisation and Integration'], in J. Tøssebro (ed.), *Integrering och Inkludering*, Lund: Lund Academic Press.

Tideman, M., and Tøssebro, J. (2002), 'A Comparison of the Living Conditions of Intellectually Disabled People in Norway and Sweden', *Scandinavian Journal of Disability Research*, vol. 4, 23–42.

Tilley, E. (1998), 'A History of Mencap, 1970–2000' (Open University Unpublished Phd thesis).

Tilley, E. (2006), 'Resistance in Mencap's History', in Mitchell (ed.), *Exploring Experiences of Advocacy by People with Learning Difficulties*, pp. 128–41.

Tilley, E. (forthcoming), Research for PhD thesis 'Advocacy Organisations for People with Learning Difficulties'

Titmuss, R. (1959), 'Community Care as Challenge', *The Times*, 12 May, 11.

Titmuss, R. M. (1961), 'Care – or Cant?', *Spectator*, 17 March, 354–6.

Titmuss, R. M. (1962), 'Community Care – Fact or Fiction?', in Freeman and Farndale (eds), *Trends in the Mental Health Services*, pp. 221–5.

Tizard, J. (1960), 'Residential Care of Mentally Handicapped Children', *British Medical Journal*, vol. i, 1041–6.

Tizard, J. (1964), *Community Services for the Mentally Handicapped*, Oxford: Oxford University Press.

Tizard, J., and Grad, J. C. (1961), *The Mentally Handicapped and their Families: A Social Survey*, Oxford: Oxford University Press.

Tizard, J., and O'Connor, N. (1952), 'The Occupational Adaptation of High-Grade Mental Defectives', *Lancet*, vol. ii, 620–3.

Tizard, J., Sinclair, I., and Clarke, R. V. G. (eds) (1975), *Varieties of Residential Experience*, London: Routledge & Kegan Paul.

Todd, S., and Shearn, J. (1997), 'Family Dilemmas and Secrets: Parents' Disclosure of Information to Their Adult Offspring with Learning Disabilities', *Disability and Society*, vol. 12, no. 3, 341–66.

Todd, S., Shearn, J., Felce, D., and Beyer, S. (1993), 'Reflecting on Change: Consumer Views of the Impact of the All Wales Strategy', *Mental Handicap*, vol. 21, 128–36.

Tonkiss, F., and Passey, A. (1999), 'Trust, Confidence and Voluntary Organisations: Between Values and Institutions', *Sociology*, vol. 33, no. 2, 257–74.

Torjman, S. (1988), *Income Insecurity: The Disability Income System in Canada*, Toronto: G. Allan Roeher Institute.

Tøssebro, J. (1992), *Institusjonsliv i Velferdsstaten. Levekår i HVPU [Institutions and the Welfare State: Living Conditions of Learning Disabled People]*, Oslo: Ad Notam Gyldendal.

Tøssebro, J. (1997), 'Family Attitudes to Deinstitutionalisation Before and After Resettlement', *Journal of Developmental and Physical Disabilities*, vol. 10, 55–72.

Tøssebro, J. (2005), 'Reflections on Living Outside: Continuity and Change in the life of "Outsiders" ', in Johnson and Traustadottir (eds), *Deinstitutionalisation and People with Intellectual Disabilities*, pp. 184–204.

Tøssebro, J., and Lundeby, H. (2002), *Statlig Reform og Kommunal Hverdag. [National Reform and Local Everyday Life: Living Conditions of People with Learning Disabilities Ten Years After]*, Trondheim: Norwegian University of Science and Technology, ISH report series no. 33.

Tøssebro, J., and Lundeby, H. (2006), 'Family Attitudes to Deinstitutionalisation: Changes During and After Reform Years in a Scandinavian Country', *Journal of Intellectual and Developmental Disabilities*, vol. 31, no. 2, 115–19.

Tøssebro, J., Aalto, M., and Brusén, P. (1996), 'Changing Ideologies and Patterns of Services: The Nordic Countries', in J. Tøssebro, A. Gustavsson and G. Dyrendahl (eds), *Intellectual Disabilities in the Nordic Welfare States*, Kristiansand: Norwegian Academic Press, pp. 45–66.

Townsend, P. (1962), *The Last Refuge: A Survey of Residential Institutions and Homes for the Aged in England and Wales*, London: Routledge and Kegan Paul.

Townsend, P. (1969), 'Forward: Social Planning for the Mentally Handicapped', in Morris, *Put Away*, pp. xi–xxxiii.

Traustadottir, R., and Johnson, K. (eds) (2000), *Women with Intellectual Disabilities: Finding a Place in the World*, London: Jessica Kingsley.

Tredgold, A. F. (1908), *Mental Deficiency*, London: Balliere, Tindall & Cox.

Tredgold, A. F. (1909), 'The Feeble-Minded – A Social Danger', *Eugenics Review*, vol. 1, 97–104.

Trent, J. W. Jr (1994), *Inventing the Feeble Mind: A History of Mental Retardation in the United States*, Berkeley, CA: University of California Press.

Unsworth, C. (1987), *The Politics of Mental Health Legislation*, Oxford: Clarendon Press.

Vasey, S. (2004) 'Disability Culture: The Story so Far' in J. Swain *et al.* (eds), *Disabling Barriers – Enabling Environments* (2nd edn), London: Sage.

Viewpoint (2005), 'Older Carers Urged to Plan for the Future', *Viewpoint*, May, 18–19.

Walker, A. (ed.) (1982), *Community Care, The Family, The State and Social Policy*, Oxford: Blackwell.

Walker, A., and Walker, C. (1998), 'Normalisation and "Normal" Ageing: The Social Construction of Dependency Among Older People with Learning Difficulties', *Disability and Society*, vol. 13, no. 1, 125–42.

Wallace, J. (1991), *Pleasant Creek Training Centre: Report to the Director General Community Services Victoria*, Melbourne: Victorian Government Printing Service.

Walmsley, J. (1994), 'Learning Disability: Overcoming the Barriers?', in S. French (ed.), *On Equal Terms: Working with Disabled People*, London: Butterworth-Heinemann, pp. 148–60.

Walmsley, J. (1995a), 'Life History Interviews with People with Learning Disabilities', *Oral History*, vol. 23, no. 1, 71–7.

Walmsley, J. (1995b), 'Gender, Caring and Learning Disability' (Open University Unpublished PhD thesis).

Walmsley, J. (1997), 'Telling the History of Learning Disability from Local Sources', in Atkinson, Jackson and Walmsley (eds), *Forgotten Lives*, pp. 83–94.

Walmsley, J. (2000a), 'Straddling Boundaries: The Changing Roles of Voluntary Organisations, 1913–1959' in Brigham *et al.* (eds), *Crossing Boundaries*, pp. 103–22.

Walmsley, J. (2000b), 'Women and the Mental Deficiency Act of 1913: Citizenship, Sexuality and Regulation', *British Journal of Learning Disabilities*, vol. 28, no. 2, 65–70.

Walmsley, J. (2001), 'Normalisation, Emancipatory Research and Learning Disability', *Disability and Society*, vol. 16, no. 2, 187–205.

Walmsley, J. (2002), 'Principles and Types of Advocacy' in B. Gray and R. Jackson (eds), *Advocacy and Learning Disability*, London: Jessica Kingsley, pp. 24–31.

Walmsley, J. (2005), 'Institutionalisation: A Historical Perspective', in Johnson and Traustadottir (eds), *Deinstitutionalization and People with Intellectual Disabilities*, pp. 50–65.

Walmsley, J., and Johnson, K. (2003), *Inclusive Research with People with Learning Disabilities: Past, Present and Futures*, London: Jessica Kingsley.

Walmsley, J., and Rolph, S. (2001), 'The Development of Community Care for People with Learning Difficulties 1913 to 1946', *Critical Social Policy*, vol. 21, no. 1, 59–80.

Walmsley, J., Atkinson, D., and Rolph, S. (1999), 'Community Care and Mental Deficiency 1913 to 1945', in Bartlett and Wright (eds), *Outside the Walls of the Asylum*, pp. 181–203.

Ward, L. (1989), 'For Better, For Worse?', in Brechin and Walmsley (eds), *Making Connections*, pp. 188–98.

Ward, L. (1998) (ed) *Innovations in Advocacy and Empowerment for People with Intellectual Disabilities*, Chorley: Lisieux Hall.

Waterhouse, L., and McGhee, J. (2002), 'Social Work in Scotland: After Devolution' in Payne and Shardlow (eds), *Social Work in the British Isles*, pp. 131–55.

Watson, J. (1970a), 'A Lingering Nightmare: Illinois Care for the Retarded Still Falls Short', *Chicago Sun-Times*, vol. XXVI, 26 July, sec. 2, 1–3.

Watson, J. (1970b), 'A House of Horror for State's Retarded', *Chicago Sun-Times*, 27 July, 52.

Webster, C. (1988), *The Health Services Since the War: Volume 1: Problems of Health Care: The National Health Service Before 1957*, London: HMSO.

Webster, C. (1994), 'Conservatives and Consensus: The Politics of the National Health Service, 1951–64', in A. Oakley and S. Williams (eds), *The Politics of the Welfare State*, London: UCL Press, pp. 54–73.

Webster, C. (1996), *The Health Services Since the War: Volume II: Government and Health Care: The British National Health Service 1958–1979*, London: HMSO.

Webster, C. (2002), *The National Health Service: A Political History* (2nd edn), Oxford: Oxford University Press.

Weisbrod, B. A. (1988), *The Non-Profit Economy*, Cambridge, MA: Harvard University Press.

Welshman, J. (1996), 'In Search of the "Problem Family": Public Health and Social Work in England and Wales, 1940–70', *Social History of Medicine*, vol. 9, no. 3, 447–65.

Welshman, J. (1999a), 'Rhetoric and Reality: Community Care in England and Wales, 1948–74', in Bartlett and Wright (eds), *Outside the Walls of the Asylum*, pp. 204–26.

Welshman, J. (1999b), 'Evacuation, Hygiene, and Social Policy: the *Our Towns* Report of 1943', *Historical Journal*, vol. 42, no. 3, 781–807.

Welshman, J. (2000), *Municipal Medicine: Public Health in Twentieth Century Britain*, Oxford and Bern: Peter Lang AG.

Welshman, J. (2005), 'Hospital Provision, Resource Allocation, and the Early National Health Service: The Sheffield Regional Hospital Board, 1947–74', in M. Pelling and S. Mandelbrote (eds), *The Practice of Reform in Health, Medicine, and Science 1500–2000: Essays for Charles Webster*, Aldershot: Ashgate, pp. 279–301.

Welshman, J. (2006a), 'Inside the Walls of the Hostel, 1940–74', in Dale and Melling (eds), *Mental Illness and Learning Disability Since 1850: Finding a place for Mental Disorder in the United Kingdom*, pp. 200–23.

Welshman, J. (2006b), 'The Concept of the Unemployable', *Economic History Review*, vol. LIX, no. 3, 578–606.

Wendell, S. (1996), *The Rejected Body*, London: Routledge.

Wertheimer, A. (1998), *Citizen Advocacy: A Powerful Partnership*, London: CAIT.

'Where Toys Are Locked Away' (1965), *Christian Century*, vol. LXXXII, 29 September, 1179.

Whitaker, S. (2004), 'Hidden Learning Disability', *British Journal of Learning Disabilities*, vol. 32, no. 3, 39–43.

White Paper no. 88, 1966–67, *On the Development of Services for Disabled People*, Oslo.

Williams, C. J. (1984), *A History of the Ontario Ministry of Community and Social Services: 1930–1980*, Toronto: Ministry of Community and Social Services.

Williams, P., and Atkinson, D. (1989), 'Networks', Workbook 2, *K262 Learning Disability: Changing Perspectives*, Milton Keynes: Open University.

Williams, P., and Shoultz, B. (1982), *We Can Speak for Ourselves*, London: Souvenir Press.

Williston, W. B. (1971), *Present Arrangements for the Care and Supervision of Mentally Retarded Persons in Ontario*, Report to the Ontario Minister of Health.

Wilmot, F., and Saul, P. (1998), *A Breath of Fresh Air: Birmingham Open-Air Schools, 1911–1970*, Chichester: Phillimore.

Wolfensberger, W. (1972), *The Principle of Normalisation in Human Services*, Toronto: National Institute on Mental Retardation.

Wolfensberger, W. (1973), 'Citizen Advocacy for the Handicapped, Impaired and Disadvantaged: An Overview', in W. Wolfensberger and H. Zauha (eds), *Citizen Advocacy and Protective Services for the Impaired and Handicapped*, Toronto: National Institute on Mental Retardation.

Wolfensberger, W. (1975), *The Origins and Nature of our Institutional Models*, Syracuse: Human Policy Press.

Wolfensberger, W. (1983), 'Social Role Valorization: A Proposed New Term for the Principle of Normalization', *Mental Retardation*, vol. 21, no. 6, 234–9.

Wolfensberger, W. (1984), *Voluntary Association On Behalf of Societally Devalued and/or Handicapped People*, Toronto: National Institute on Mental Retardation.

Wolfensberger, W., and Tullman, S. (1989), 'A Brief Outline of the Principle of Normalisation', in Brechin and Walmsley (eds), *Making Connections*, pp. 211–19.

Woodring, P. (1962), 'Slow Learners', *Saturday Review*, vol. XLV, 17 February, 53–4.

Wright, F. J. Jr (1947), *Out of Sight, Out of Mind*, Philadelphia, PA: National Mental Health Foundation.

Wright, D. (1998), 'Familial Care of Idiot Children in Victorian England', in P. Horden and R. Smith (eds), *The Locus of Care: Families, Communities, Institutions and the Provision of Welfare since Antiquity*, London: Routledge, pp. 176–97.

Wright, K., Haycox, A., and Leedham, I. (1994), *Evaluating Community Care*, Buckingham: Open University Press.

Zahn, G. C. (1946a), 'State School Unnatural, Mistreats Children', *Catholic Worker*, vol. XIII, July/August, 5–7.

Zahn, G. C. (1946b), 'Slaves or Patients?: Rosewood and Enforced Labor', *Catholic Worker*, vol. XIII, September, 6.

Zahn, G. C. (1946c), 'Abandon Hope', *Catholic Worker*, vol. XIII, October, 4–6.

Zarfas, D. (1976), 'Ontario', in Kugel and Shearer (eds), *Changing Patterns in Residential Services for the Mentally Retarded*, pp. 267–75.

Zaslow, J. (2005), 'The Graduates: What Happens after Young Disabled Adults Leave School', *Wall Street Journal*, vol. CCXLVI, 29 December, p. D4.

Index